Practicing Psychology

in Hospitals and Other

Health Care Facilities

Practicing Psychology

in Hospitals and Other

Health Care Facilities

AMERICAN PSYCHOLOGICAL ASSOCIATION

PRACTICE DIRECTORATE

AMERICAN PSYCHOLOGICAL ASSOCIATION

WASHINGTON, DC

> *Important:* Depending on a psychologist's training and background, some
> sections of this document will be more pertinent and useful than others.
> Please note that this document is for informational purposes only and does
> not represent American Psychological Association policy.

Published by
American Psychological Association
750 First Street, NE
Washington, DC 20002

Copies may be ordered from
APA Order Department
P.O. Box 92984
Washington, DC 20090-2984

Typeset in Century by EPS Group Inc., Easton, MD

Printer: United Book Press, Baltimore, MD
Cover designer: Kachergis Book Design, Pittsboro, NC
Technical/production editor: Tanya Y. Alexander

Library of Congress Cataloging-in-Publication Data
Practicing psychology in hospitals and other health care facilities /
  by the American Psychological Association Practice Directorate.
      p.   cm.
   Includes bibliographical references and index.
   ISBN 1-55798-491-3 (pbk.)
   1. Clinical psychology—Practice.   2. Psychology—Practice.
3. Hospitals—Medical staff—Clinical privileges.   I. American
Psychological Association.
Practice Directorate.
RC467.95.P678   1998
616.89'0068—dc21   97-51278
                                                              CIP

Printed in the United States of America
First Edition

Contents

Preface

The purpose of this consolidated and updated text is to provide information and strategies that will help promote more effective utilization of psychologists within hospitals and other health care facilities.[1] It is directed to psychologists in independent practice, in public service, and in private sector employment who wish to gain access to and recognized standing in hospitals to render professional services whether they are working as salaried staff or on a fee-for-service or contract basis. It is intended to identify many of the obstacles that have restricted psychologists' access and full professional participation in hospital and other health facility settings and to serve as a blueprint for overcoming these obstacles.

Treating people's psychological problems sometimes involves hospitalization as well as outpatient treatment. The interest of the public demands that all appropriate resources be available to assist in the diagnosis, prevention, treatment, and amelioration of psychological problems. As independent health care providers, psychologists can take active roles in encouraging health care facilities to admit psychologists to membership on organized staffs, with full participation in the governance system. This could lead to the exercise of clinical privileges and professional responsibilities consistent with the scope of the licensure and the competence of psychologists.

This book provides information about pertinent hospital issues such as staff privileges; organized staff membership; roles for psychologists in hospitals; training for psychological work in hospitals; and the legal, legislative, and regulatory matters that have an impact on such practice. The book also suggests ways of achieving appropriate recognition in status, salary, and governance within the hospital setting. It is intended to provide needed information, support, and guidance to assist psychologists in beginning or enhancing health care facility–based practice. The book should stimulate discussion and action promoting the hospital practice of psychology.

The Need for Hospital Privileges

Health care services are being used in greater quantity by more people than ever before. Psychologists are trained to provide a broad range of these health care services. As a profession, psychology is represented in virtually every health care delivery system. In state and federal programs and in most communities throughout the United States, psychologists are recognized as providing needed, valuable, and cost-effective health services. There is, however, one health delivery sector in which psycholo-

---

[1] Throughout this book, the term *hospital* should be understood to also encompass "other health care facilities" where appropriate.

gists' full participation has not yet been as widely realized as it should be, namely, hospitals.

Psychologists' patients may be persons with severe mental disorders who need 24-hour residential acute care. They could also be patients with a wide range of acute and chronic medical conditions, often manifesting concurrent psychological problems, such as panic or anxiety states following an unexpected heart attack, progressive depression associated with the need for continued renal dialysis, neuromuscular retraining following a stroke, pain management following an accident, or the need for control of enuresis or encopresis among some children and older persons. This is just a brief illustration of the range of medical conditions in which psychological intervention has been proven to be effective both clinically and costwise. If not addressed, such problems may seriously impede recovery from or stabilization of the patient's medical condition. With psychological intervention there is substantial potential for earlier recovery, adoption of necessary lifestyle change, and reduction of total health care costs. Indeed, as Pallak, Cummings, Dörken, and Henke (1994) showed in studying the impact of psychological intervention in a Medicaid population, the greatest cost savings were achieved among those patients with a chronic medical disease, replicating an earlier finding by Schlesinger, Mumford, Patrick, and Sharfstein (1983).

To assure appropriate and continuing attention to the treatment needs of these patients, psychologists must have direct access to hospitals and other health care facilities. This is extremely important, for not only is the patient better served, but also the facility itself benefits from exposure to the wide range of health management and professional skills of professional psychology.

As independent practitioners and members of a hospital's organized staff (or other facility staff organizations), psychologists are better positioned to influence institutional policy and services and to provide continuity of patient care. Membership in the organized medical and professional staff allows them collegial standing with physicians and parity in decisions that affect the institution. Because psychologists have a different perspective—a behavioral health perspective—their influence on institutional policy can promote the provision of a broader range of effective, noninvasive, and often less expensive health services. Staff membership allows psychologists to participate in clinical research and professional training, budget planning, and facility clinical activities; to influence hiring and promotion practices; and to help improve contract arrangements (Copeland, 1980).

Although many psychologists are trained in hospitals, extensive control of the institutional health services of this country by physicians has often prevented psychologists' participation in an appropriate and consistent way. Consequently, psychologists have traditionally been more associated with office-based practice. Moving to a health care facility environment may be unsettling; customs, practice, and even the language are often unfamiliar. Other hospital professional staff may be unaware of the role psychologists can play in general health care delivery. Occasionally,

there can be internecine battles regarding clinical authority that may neu-
tralize psychologists' effectiveness. A sometimes rigid hierarchical organization can even dictate social amenities such as the allocation of parking
spaces, acquisition of supplies, and where lunch can be purchased! Complex issues that cross the boundaries of psychology, other professions, hospital policy, local customs, regulatory agencies, and state law confront psychologists in a hospital environment.

Typically, state psychology practice statutes are silent about the site
of practice; that is, licensing laws focus on the types of services psychologists provide, not the location in which they are provided. Then, too,
changes in the standards adopted by the Joint Commission on Accreditation of Healthcare Organizations for hospitals and other health care facilities over the past decade, and the broadened direct recognition by third-
party payers under state insurance laws, have strengthened psychologists'
efforts to demonstrate to legislators and to hospital administrators that
psychologists can provide needed quality services independently in hospital settings. Unfortunately, interprofessional rivalry has often made this
task arduous. For some health plans, psychologists have been excluded
from medical "peer" review activities traditionally dominated by physicians (e.g., current Civilian Health and Medical Program of the Uniformed
Services regulations require all inpatient peer reviews to be completed by
physicians regardless of who provides the service). Thus, psychologists are
often subject to controls imposed by disciplines with little or no understanding of psychological practice. Because of such impediments and the lack of
clear state legislation, psychologists are often still denied status as independent health care practitioners or as active staff members in a hospital.

Evaluating Psychology's Current Status in Hospitals

Hospital privileges for psychologists are actually part of a continuous ev-
olutionary process. The acquisition of hospital staff membership is only
the beginning of this process (Dörken, 1983). Because credentialing in hospitals has been one basis for health care recognition of the independent
practice of psychology, hospitals can have an important impact on determining the profession's stature in other settings and its place in future
health policy initiatives.

Health care delivery systems are being forced to change by the rising
cost of care, by mandated cost-containment efforts and the growing de-
mand for improved quality of health care, and by the progressive industrialization of health care. Organized health provider groups are burgeon-
ing, including preferred provider organizations, exclusive provider
organizations, independent practice associations, physician practice management organizations, health maintenance organizations, and hospital-
based networks with satellite outpatient clinics. Established physician and
other professional practices are being bought out or assimilated into practice organizations that compete for health care delivery markets in which
their services are provided under contract. Medical staff membership

makes psychologists' professional services more valuable to a managed care organization because it enables (although it does not guarantee) access not simply to hospital inpatient services but also to all services within the hospital's ambit, while making the psychologist more broadly useful.

Many evolving forms of health care service delivery are often dominated by physicians. The inroads psychologists have made in achieving recognition cannot be taken for granted; psychologists must safeguard and advance these accomplishments continuously. The health care marketplace is changing so rapidly that legislators and administrators may not keep pace with the changes. Practicing psychologists, by active participation and leadership (rather than opposition to change), can play a critical role in educating these decision makers and thus ensure their own presence and survival in the health care arena.

In addition to the historical reasons for the psychologists' need to secure hospital privileges, there is a practical reason: The transfer of control over patient treatment when a patient is admitted to an inpatient setting is inefficient and interrupts the continuity of care. Requiring a patient to change clinicians not only is disruptive and traumatic but also can add to the cost and length of treatment required. In this time of cutting costs and shortening hospital stays, psychologists can play a major role in the hospital setting, particularly if they possess the hospital privileges that will ensure continuity and efficiency of patient care.

Psychologists interested in hospital practice must be prepared to contribute to the facility and to the community at large. They will be asked, and are strongly encouraged, to serve on facility committees and to work with community groups, thereby enhancing the service delivery system by providing a psychological perspective. By broadening the range and quality of its health services with psychologists' services, a hospital can provide optimal patient care to the community it serves.

Acknowledgments

Part I of this book was conceived and initiated by the American Psychological Association's (APA's) Committee on Professional Practice (COPP) of the Board of Professional Affairs (BPA). It was originally published as *A Hospital Practice Primer for Psychologists* (APA, 1985). Members of the committee at that time included Jean Balinky, EdD (chair, 1984); Faith Tanney, PhD (chair, 1983); Jacob Chwast, PhD; Thomas Hefele, PhD; Thomas Overcast, PhD; Cass Turner, PhD; Norma P. Simon, EdD; Jarold Niven, PhD; and R. Mark Mays, PhD. Much of the text was written and developed by the COPP Subcommittee on Hospital Practice, which convened in December 1983. Members of that subcommittee included Thomas Hefele, PhD, chair; Richard Cohen, PhD; Norman Karl, PhD; C. Eric Levy, PhD; Samuel Mayhugh, PhD; Robert J. Resnick, PhD; Judith Steller, PhD; and Anita Washington, PhD; with subsequent consultation by Herbert Dörken, PhD, while a member of COPP (1986–1988), the Committee on Employment and Human Resources (1991–1993), and BPA (1994–1996). In addition, various state psychological associations and individual APA members shared their own manuscripts on hospital practice. APA central office support was provided by Professional Practice Program staff members Patricia J. Aletky, Bev Hitchins, Sharon Scott, Rizalina Mendiola, and Elizabeth Cullen, JD, MPA, and State Associations Program staff members Mark Ginsberg, PhD, and William Buklad.

Part II of this book also was conceived and initiated by COPP. It was originally published as *Hospital Practice: Advocacy Issues* (APA, 1988). Members of the committee at that time included David H. Reilly, EdD (chair, 1987); R. Mark Mays, PhD (chair, 1986); Thomas J. Hefele, PhD (chair, 1985); Robert J. Resnick, PhD; Herbert Dörken, PhD; Norma P. Simon, EdD; Jarold R. Niven, PhD; G. Rita Dudley, PhD; and Hannah R. Hirsh. Much of the original text was written and developed by the COPP Subcommittee on Hospital Practice II, which convened twice in 1985. Members of that subcommittee included Robert J. Resnick, PhD, chair; Richard M. Cohen, PhD; Anthony D. Sciara, PhD; Leonard W. Allen, PhD; Ted Brown, PhD; Jonathan W. Cummings, PhD; Eugene C. Stammeyer, PhD; and C. Eric Levy, PhD. APA Central Office support was provided at that time by Professional Affairs staff members Bev Hitchins; Patricia J. Aletky; Russ Newman, PhD, JD; Rizalina Mendiola; and Mary Lisa Debraggio. Other APA staff who provided helpful guidance included Mary Uyeda and Donna Daley.

Part III of this book was conceived and initiated by the BPA. Members of the committee at that time included J. Gilbert Benedict, PhD; Bruce E. Bennett, PhD; Allen C. Carter, PhD; Richard M. Cohen, PhD; Herbert Dörken, PhD; Lorraine Eyde, PhD; Mark S. Goldman, PhD; Leonard J. Haas, PhD; Joseph C. Kobos, PhD (chair, 1994); Rodney Lowman, PhD (chair, 1993); Deborah Tharinger, PhD; and Melba Vasquez, PhD. Much of the text was written and developed by the BPA Task Force on Quality Assurance, which was established in 1990. Members of the task force included Thomas Grundle, PhD, and Cynthia White, PsyD. Additional contributors included Thomas Cook, PhD, and Geoffrey Porosoff, PhD. APA Central Office support was provided by the Practice Directorate's Office of Legal and Regulatory Affairs staff member Elizabeth A. Cullen, JD, MPA.

The extensive revisions, updates, additions, and annotated references required to meld these three parts into this edition were provided by Herbert Dörken, PhD; John R. Erbeck, PhD; Charles Faltz, PhD; and Practice Directorate staff member Cherie Jones, JD.

Practicing Psychology in Hospitals and Other Health Care Facilities

Part I _____

Hospital Practice for Psychologists

1 _____

Psychologists' Roles and Responsibilities in Hospital Practice

This chapter describes the variety of roles and responsibilities psychologists have in hospitals and other residential treatment settings commensurate with their individual training and experience and state law. In fact, the types of psychological services offered in these facilities vary tremendously according to the mission of the particular facility, the skills and expertise of the psychologist, and the needs of the patient population. The functions delineated in this chapter serve only as examples of these services; clearly, the list is not exhaustive.

Psychological Assessment

Psychological assessment is frequently equated with psychological testing. However, most psychologists design their assessment approach according to the particular setting, its mission, and the problems and needs of the person being evaluated. The diagnostic interview and a review of previous records and additional sources of data collected by other mental health and medical practitioners, obtained in either a group or individual setting, are probably the most common components of psychological assessments. Another frequently used approach is a behavioral appraisal during which the psychologist observes the patient in a variety of settings, noting the skills or lack of skills demonstrated, the frequency of particular behaviors, reinforcement contingencies, and other necessary information for the planning of behavioral interventions. In addition, when necessary and appropriate, such as with individuals who are developmentally disabled, psychologists will interview caretakers and other knowledgeable parties about the individual's adaptive functions. Finally, psychologists will determine what type of testing (e.g., cognitive, educational, vocational, or personality), if any, is necessary to address specific questions about the individual.

Treatment Planning: Psychologists as Team Leaders, Team Members, and Team Consultants

Psychologists participate in the multidisciplinary treatment planning process as team leaders, team members, and consultants. The task of the team leader often involves integrating and assimilating information from all members of the treatment team or may entail coordinating and developing a comprehensive treatment plan for the patient. Treatment planning may address more traditional forms of treatment, such as psychotherapy, and/or detailed and specific recommendations for behavioral management. The task of a team member may involve implementing the treatment plan. The consultative role may involve attending the treatment planning meeting and verbally summarizing the psychological assessment or making specific recommendations regarding treatment plans on the basis of information provided by the treatment team.

Clinical Interventions

Psychologists provide a wide variety of clinical interventions, including individual, group, family, and behavior therapy; behavioral consultations for health-related problems; biofeedback; psychoeducational group therapy; and a variety of other techniques. In the area of behavior therapy alone, psychologists have been active in pain management, psychosocial rehabilitation (e.g., social skills training), compliance with medication regimens, and the development of alternatives to unnecessary sole reliance on restraint/seclusion and the psychotropic medication in the management of violence.

Admission, Diagnosis, Treatment, and Discharge

Psychologists increasingly are assuming responsibility for the admission, diagnosis, treatment, and discharge of patients in hospitals and other residential treatment facilities. Many of these tasks historically have been performed by physicians. Psychologists conduct patient evaluations, coordinate and lead patient conferences, recommend treatments at prescribed levels of intensity, arrange for patients to be discharged, and thereby bear ultimate responsibility for the care they provide.

Scientific Research

Psychologists in hospitals and other residential treatment facilities are actively engaged in scientific research. As a group, they are specifically trained for this; in particular, those psychologists with doctoral degrees are assumed to have engaged in original research as part of their graduate training. The scope of their research activities includes the design and conduct of a wide variety of research projects, such as case studies, treatment efficacy or outcome studies, program evaluation, and formal clinical projects that are either externally or internally funded.

Management and Administration

Psychologists can be found at all levels of management and administration in hospitals and other residential treatment settings. Increasingly, psychologists have come to serve as chief executive officers and directors and heads of units, departments, or divisions within these facilities. They fulfill these administrative and leadership roles for both inpatient and outpatient services in areas such as neuropsychology, rehabilitation, mental health, pediatrics, occupational health, and emergency care. Some also direct hospice programs, alcohol and drug abuse services, gerontological services, and behavioral medicine programs for the treatment of such problems as eating disorders, sleep disorders, pain management, and biofeedback.

Psychologists are also taking on leadership responsibilities in both the hospital governance structure and personnel programs. A growing number of psychologists have acquired full medical or professional staff membership, are assuming committee duties, and increasingly are running for elected staff positions, such as chief of the medical or professional staff. In addition, psychologists are involving themselves with personnel training services, such as continuing education, residency training of psychologists, physicians and nurses, staff development, and employee assistance programs.[2]

---

[2]As of 1996, the Council for the National Register of Health Service Providers in Psychology listed over 2,100 registrants with verified hospital staff membership.

2 _____

Training Psychologists for Hospital Practice

Many psychologists are already qualified to work in hospitals by virtue of their graduate education, specialized training, and experience. It may be desirable for more psychologists to get additional training to function effectively in the hospital setting. Of course, it should be kept in mind that psychologists practicing in hospitals will be licensed in accordance with the statutes and administrative regulations of their respective states. Licensure, in general, requires a doctoral degree in psychology, successful completion of a comprehensive licensing examination, and 2 years of supervised experience. Beyond these requirements, some psychologists will complete specialty examinations conducted by the American Board of Professional Psychology and by other boards that confer the diplomate status.

Accredited Graduate Education and Training in Psychology

Typically, in accredited doctoral psychology programs, students complete a wide variety of course work that has relevance to the practice of psychology in hospital settings. In addition to academic courses, requirements include practica and clerkships in which students gain experience with qualified supervisors in applied settings. For most students, graduate training relevant to hospital practice usually includes the following subjects.

Physiological Psychology, Neuropsychology, and Psychopharmacology

These courses are concerned with the biological bases of behavior and are directly relevant to issues of mental health and mental illness. In particular, knowledge about the role of brain dysfunction in the etiology of cognitive and behavioral disturbances is critical in hospital practice, both for rehabilitative and therapeutic purposes and to provide knowledge about the functional origin of some medical problems. Courses in physiological psychology include training in biofeedback and in psychophysiological assessment.

Developmental Psychology

Courses in this area provide an understanding of development over the life span. Psychologists' particular knowledge about physical, cognitive, and emotional development enables them to bring effective resources to the treatment of people in all stages of the life cycle, from infancy through old age, including gender differences.

Cognitive Psychology

Training in this area enables psychologists to evaluate the perceptual, cognitive, and memory capabilities of patients and to make specific recommendations for remedial treatment of impaired functions. These recommendations enable the treatment staff to assist the patient in using his or her internal and external resources to gain from specialized treatment. Diagnostic questions can also be clarified more expeditiously with an understanding of the skills and limitations of a particular patient.

Personality

Assessment of psychological functioning requires a thorough understanding of normal and abnormal personality theory and research. Such information is critical to the delivery of individualized treatment, both medical and psychological.

Statistics and Research Design

An essential requirement of training in graduate psychology programs is 1 year of advanced statistics and research design. The skills provided by such courses are applicable to the process of treatment evaluation, hospital based general research, and large-scale testing and assessment programs in hospitals.

Social Psychology

Illness, as well as treatment, always has a social context. Social psychology courses sensitize students to the ways in which cultural subgroups respond to stress, illness, and treatment approaches and to the value of family and social support systems in recovery. In addition, knowledge of social psychology contributes to an understanding of the hospital itself as social system.

Community Psychology

The study of community psychology provides an awareness of the impact of communities on the creation of both physical and psychological problems and on intervention and treatment. An essential focus of community psychology is that the community is the unit of concern, that constructive change in the community can alleviate some personal and family problems and facilitate adaptations. Dysfunctional communities jeopardize personal and social stability. Community psychology courses also sensitize psychology students to issues of illness prevention, minority group differences, and cultural differences.

General Psychological, Intellectual, and Personality Assessment

Psychologists in hospital settings are often called on to complete the psychological assessment of general medical patients, psychiatric patients, and patients in other specialty departments such as pediatrics, internal medicine, and neurology. Graduate students in psychology are usually required to take at least several courses that include practica in assessment.

Individual Interventions

Courses and practica in various systems of intervention that are designed to effect behavioral change can be applied to both general medical and psychiatric patients.

Group Interventions

Course work and practicum experience that are designed to effect group behavioral change can be applied in working with both general medical and psychiatric patients as well as to the organizational structure and programs of the hospital and any satellite community outpatient services.

Organizational Development

As part of programs in clinical psychology, counseling psychology, and industrial/organizational psychology, organizational development courses provide both theory and applied experience in the functioning of organizations as systems. Such skills can be helpful to psychologists in working with hospital administrators and other professionals.

Forensic Psychology

Courses in forensic psychology provide psychologists with knowledge and skills for making decisions regarding a variety of legal matters such as civil commitment, criminal justice, parental custody, competence to stand trial, and ability to give informed consent.

Internships

Psychology internships typically include both inpatient and outpatient experiences with emotionally disordered or physically impaired populations. Supervised training in diagnosis, treatment, record keeping, patient management, and consultation–liaison to a diverse population (e.g., to medical, surgical, psychiatric, rehabilitation medical, and geriatric patients) is often available in a predoctoral internship program. Learning to understand the nuances of hospital organizational structure and the interrelationship of health care professionals may be a valuable part of the internship year. The predoctoral internship offers a broad range of experiences with diverse patient populations to prepare the psychologist for the multiple roles he or she may assume in a hospital-based practice.

In the event that a psychologist has not had the relevant hospital-based training, it is incumbent on him or her to comply with APA standards in acquiring the appropriate skills and the necessary postdoctoral supervised experience. (See "Ethical Principles of Psychologists and Code of Conduct" [APA, 1992] and "General Guidelines for Providers of Psychological Services" [APA, 1987].)

Postdoctoral Training

Beyond the core curriculum, practica, clerkships, and internships, many psychologists have completed postdoctoral training that further qualifies them to work in a hospital setting. Postdoctoral study in areas such as pediatrics, behavioral medicine, and neuropsychology are examples of specialized training that are valuable assets to a hospital practice. Furthermore, continuing education is another avenue by which psychologists expand their knowledge and skills relevant to hospital practice.

What is described here is essentially a framework for basic training. If their training and experience are incomplete, psychologists interested in hospital practice can obtain the appropriate training and experience through internships, postdoctoral residencies, or continuing education courses. These experiences should be oriented toward psychology practice that is hospital based and that includes experience in multidisciplinary team planning. Those interested in pursuing training in illness management and health enhancement practice may consult, among other resources, the APA Division of Health Psychology.

3

The Hospital Organization: Psychological Services in a Hospital Context

Although psychologists' expertise is in providing psychological services, they may not be knowledgeable about the hospital organization within which these services can be provided. In fact, for those not trained in a hospital setting, it can seem to be an alien or intimidating social system or subculture. The purpose of this section is to address the need of many psychologists working in hospitals to better understand this environment, so that they might function more effectively in this special health care setting. This section provides (a) a description of the structure and operation of a hospital, (b) a review of the structures and functions of hospital staffs, and (c) a summary of some of the key issues that psychologists need to understand as they develop working roles in hospital settings. The following is adapted, in large part, from the work of Anthony Sciara (1983).

The Typical Organization and Operation of a Hospital

Board of Directors or Board of Trustees

One system of authority and responsibility in a hospital is the board of directors or board of trustees. Whether the hospital is private or public, for profit or nonprofit, there will be a governing board of some type. That board, whether it consists of the owners or of a board of trustees, has the obligation for maintaining the hospital at a certain level of quality and for providing certain types of services. The governing board oversees all hospital operations and promulgates policies and procedures. Theoretically, board members are not engaged in day-to-day activities of the hospital; they are engaged in major policy- and decision-making tasks.

The governing board is thus accountable for the running of the hospital—to the community, in the case of a public hospital, or to the owners, in the case of a private, for-profit hospital. In either case, there are certain goals that have been established by the hospital to fulfill the needs of the community, the patients, and the owners, or the individuals for whom the hospital is being held in trust. It is these board members who are ultimately responsible for all that occurs in the hospital, and these individuals may be held jointly and separately responsible for the activities of the hospital. Their responsibility is obviously a paramount one, and one to be taken seriously.

Hospital Administration

One line of authority reporting to the governing board is the administration of the hospital. The administration comprises those individuals who are directly responsible for the day-to-day operation of the hospital. Administrative personnel are responsible for the nonclinical aspects of patient care, which include housekeeping, dietary, medical records, maintenance, and clerical. The administration is characteristically responsible directly to the board of directors or board of trustees for ensuring that the day-to-day activities of the hospital are in concert with the goals set by them.

This is often a difficult position for both the administrator and the clinical staff because those things that affect the quality of hospital care are dependent on both administrative and clinical efficiency in the use of costly resources. Although these are major concerns of the administrator, the clinicians may perceive them differently. Resolving conflicts between administrative and clinical personnel is essential and requires sensitive handling. In the modern hospital, a rapidly changing health care environment places a great deal of responsibility on the hospital administrator for keeping the hospital financially viable.

Organized Medical or Professional Staff

A second line of authority and responsibility in a hospital is the medical or professional staff. The medical staff is responsible for all clinical care within the hospital. As such, the medical staff is responsible for reporting to the governing board on the current status of the clinical staff and about the quality of care offered by the hospital. The medical staff functions pursuant to the written bylaws and rules of the hospital. It is the responsibility of the medical staff and the administration to work jointly in running the hospital from both an administrative and a clinical standpoint, so that the goals of the board are met and the quality of patient care is appropriate. It is the medical staff that has the primary responsibility for the way in which individual psychologists and physicians practice within the hospital setting.

Laws, Bylaws, Rules, and Regulations

The laws, bylaws, rules, and regulations (e.g., for Medicaid, Medicare, and third-party payers) to which hospitals must conform may be confusing.

These rules and regulations, however, guide practice in the hospital setting and restrict practice to certain professionals. It is important to examine each of these areas individually.

State hospital licensing laws and regulations. Each state has promulgated laws and regulations by which hospitals must abide. These laws protect consumers and hospitals and are administered by a state agency that maintains at least some interaction with hospitals. In most states, there are several sections of law that are concerned with different types of hospitals, including public, private for-profit and private nonprofit, general and specialty hospitals; skilled nursing facilities; and other types of treatment facilities. These laws often define, in a general way, who is appropriate to practice which profession in which institution. Laws may also define the types of evaluations that hospitals must perform on a regular basis to maintain licensure. In addition, state laws define the processes of voluntary and involuntary hospitalization and determine the qualifications of the professionals involved. Psychologists who wish to practice in a hospital must be very familiar with these laws.

Organized medical/professional staff. Medical/professional staff bylaws describe the roles of the professional staff of that institution. Bylaws clearly spell out the qualifications for membership on the staff, conditions and duration of appointments, categories of professional staff, and privileging for the different types of procedures that each professional staff member may perform. These bylaws usually also address quality assurance issues and due process issues in terms of work-related personnel actions. They should generally designate officers to the professional staff and the election of those officers, and they should define committees of the professional staff organization. It is generally within these bylaws that the clinical privileging of all staff and rules and regulations for practice within the hospital are defined. These rules and regulations may include documentation, care and treatment standards, admission and discharge standards, and other such matters that may affect the professional staff while they are practicing in the hospital.

Medical/professional staff bylaws must be approved by the governing board of the hospital. The bylaws are usually subject to oversight bodies such as the Joint Commission on Accreditation of Healthcare Organizations (JCAHO) and the Commission on Accreditation of Rehabilitation Facilities (CARF). The bylaws may need to be modified to provide for independent practice for psychologists in the hospital setting. Psychologists should be aware that membership on the medical staff permits voting on professional staff bylaws, whereas simply holding specific clinical privileges does not. When seeking staff membership at a hospital, it is always important for psychologists to ask for a copy of the bylaws of the professional and medical staff, which define their role when working in that institution. In fact, it is unwise for psychologists to practice without a thorough understanding of hospital bylaws and of their own legal standing in the hospital setting. Without this familiarity, psychologists risk making themselves and the hospital more vulnerable to malpractice scrutiny. Bylaws are a public document and are available to any citizen. All boards have a secretary, who must furnish or provide access to a copy when requested.

Medical staff rules. In addition to the bylaws, the medical staff may have a number of different rules by which practitioners are guided. These rules may be departmental in nature; for example, practitioners in the mental health field may have to follow the rules of an in-hospital psychology or psychiatry service or other department to which they are assigned, to comply with standards of practice. The rules may include documentation requirements, the types of orders that psychologists may write, the forms on which psychologists may write those orders, different requests that psychologists can make, and how those are defined. The difficult part about these rules is that they seem to be much more flexible and changeable than the bylaws and can change with the appointment of a new department head. It may at times be difficult to keep up with the rules in an institution. Each institution may have very different rules and obviously will have different forms. The burden of finding out about the specifics for particular institutions and how to practice within them is on the psychologist.

Joint Commission on Accreditation of Healthcare Organizations

The JCAHO is a private, nonprofit corporation that was developed for the purpose of setting standards for hospitals. This particular organization is important because as hospitals are able to meet these standards, they are then able to be reimbursed by both third-party and governmental payers for the services they provide. Without meeting these standards, most hospitals could not continue, because most third-party payers would be reluctant or unable to pay an institution that does not meet JCAHO standards.

The JCAHO standards directly affect the practice of psychology in a hospital, as is the case with standards for all other professions. The JCAHO standards define, among other things, what types of documentation must be done on patients, how the documentation must be recorded, and what things must be done with patients while they are in the hospital. These standards are very strict, and hospitals "gear up" to a high pitch before being surveyed by the JCAHO. A hospital is surveyed approximately every 3 years, and if it passes the survey, it is allowed to state that it is accredited by the JCAHO. All records of a hospital that is so accredited have been scrutinized and have been found to be appropriate to the level and quality of care that should be maintained by hospitals with high standards. Records of psychologists, too, have been scrutinized and must coincide with the types of record keeping that are necessary for JCAHO approval.

The JCAHO–State Law Interface

Organized psychology has worked through a number of direct and indirect channels to encourage hospital accreditation policy makers to make it possible for psychological skills and knowledge to begin to be more widely applied in hospital patient care. For example, after a long dialogue, in 1984 JCAHO changed its standards to permit hospitals surveyed to include on their medical staffs (in addition to physicians) "other licensed individuals permitted by law and by the hospital to provide patient care services independently in the hospital." In addition, in 1995, the *Accreditation Manual for Mental Health, Chemical Dependency, and Mental Retardation/Developmental Disabilities Services* was revised to authorize psychologists to write seclusion and restraint orders in psychiatric and substance abuse facilities, programs, and services when permitted by state law and the facility. This revision was incorporated into the *Comprehensive Accreditation Manual for Hospitals* in 1996 (JCAHO, 1996). Language in various other JCAHO standards makes clear also that psychologists must be permitted to credential and privilege other psychologists as peers, plan treatment and provide direct care, and serve as clinical leaders in hospitals (Rozensky, 1997).

Changes such as these in JCAHO policy have been largely the result of years of coordinated effort involving psychologists in the field, the APA central office, APA-affiliated state psychological associations and divisions, and public policy makers. For example, since 1988, the APA has had a representative on the Behavioral Health Professional and Technical Advisory Committee of the JCAHO. That committee oversees preparation and review of all mental health care standards for all types of health care facilities and hospitals. Thus, American psychology has an equal voice along with all health care disciplines in both setting national standards of care and in reviewing and monitoring of proposed standards of care in any and all health care organizations (Rozensky, 1997). Note, however, that JCAHO policies will apply to psychologists only to the extent that state law permits. Therefore, psychologists seeking hospital staff recognition must familiarize themselves with state hospital licensure codes and the requirements pertaining to medical staff membership as well as JCAHO guidelines.

In those states where hospital licensure codes are shown to restrict implementation of the more progressive JCAHO policies relating to staffing and privileging, amendments along the lines of those enacted in a number of states, including California, the District of Columbia, Georgia, and North Carolina, may be required. Psychologists should consult with their state association leadership in the event that corrective legislation is required. The state association leadership, in turn, should feel free to consult with the APA central office and with other state associations when an advocacy program is indicated.

Psychologists as Members of the Organized Staff

The organizational structure of the typical hospital has a wide range of subunits. There are two parallel chains of management responsibility that must be understood—the professional staff and the administrative staff, both responsible to the governing board. The responsibilities and prerogatives of each of these lines of authority vary from hospital to hospital, but psychologists should be aware of their relationship to both the administrative and professional staff as they seek privileges or provide services. These chains of command are found in each of the functional subunits of a hospital, whether the subunit be a medicosurgical ward, an inpatient mental health unit, or a pediatric inpatient service. Sensitivity to the roles and relationships among the various members of the treatment team— MDs, PhDs, nurses, administrators, physical and occupational therapists, and so forth—will increase psychologists' capacities to function effectively. What follows is a description of the organized, or medical, staff and of some of the major issues for psychologists in delineating and securing staff membership and staff privileges (see Exhibit 3.1).

There are generally two self-governance responsibilities afforded to the hospital medical staff by the governing body of the hospital:

- to monitor and evaluate the quality of patient care,
- to develop rules, regulations, and policies regarding medical staff membership and the granting, delineating, and renewal of clinical

Exhibit 3.1. Checklist for Applying for Staff Membership

_____ Obtain a copy of hospital bylaws.
_____ Determine the level of membership appropriate to qualifications.
_____ Locate necessary documents:
    _____ malpractice insurance (state requirements for coverage)
    _____ résumé
    _____ hospital experience
    _____ letters from professionals, including physicians (preferably those already on the hospital staff and familiar with work)
    _____ application letter including
        (a) request for staff membership
        (b) request for specific privileges
        (c) approximate amount of time available to practice in facility
    _____ copy of license
    _____ copy of diploma (doctoral degree)
    _____ copy of advanced certifications (e.g., American Board of Professional Psychology)
    _____ other supporting documents

privileges, which are patient care responsibilities afforded to individual practitioners.

Thus, membership on staff makes one an official and recognized part of health care provision in the hospital. Staff members may practice within the privileges that have been extended to them and within the limits imposed by institutional policies and state laws and regulations. Membership on the organized staff of hospitals can be extended to a wide range of health care providers (e.g., physicians, psychologists, dentists, and podiatrists) who meet the qualifications, standards, and requirements set forth by local individual hospital bylaws, by state laws, and by JCAHO standards.

Qualifications Required for Membership

Licensed psychologists who can document their background, experience, training, competence, adherence to APA ethical principles and those promulgated by the state, and their good reputation and ability to work with others shall usually be qualified for membership on the organized staff. Characteristically, psychologists must meet the following requirements:

- a doctoral degree in psychology from an accredited educational institution, which meets the criteria for licensure or certification in the particular state;
- at least 2 years of supervised clinical experience in an organized multidisciplinary facility licensed to provide care; and
- a license (or certificate wherever this is used) to practice in the state.

Psychologists so qualified may be eligible to join the organized or medical staff. The staff normally includes active, courtesy, consulting, honorary, and affiliate categories. The categories of staff membership are defined in the hospital bylaws and may vary from institution to institution. Typically, the medical staff is also organized by department, by clinical service, or by both. In this situation, the exercise of clinical privileges within any department or service is subject to the rules and regulations of that department or service, under the overall purview of the medical staff and the hospital. Each department or service delineates the specific privileges related to that department or service and develops criteria for recommending privileges.

Categories of Staff Membership

Active staff. The active organized staff may consist of a variety of health care providers, including psychologists, physicians, dentists, podiatrists, and others. They have the highest levels of hospital privileges and responsibilities. They regularly admit patients to the hospital, provide con-

tinuous care to their patients, and assume all the functions and responsibilities of their membership. They may be appointed to any of the various
services, such as psychology, medicine, or pediatrics; are eligible to vote
and hold office; may serve on organized staff committees; are required to
attend organized staff meetings; and may participate in teaching and service functions in the hospital, consistent with the scope of their licensure,
competence, and privileges. Historically, the active organized staff has op-
posed nonphysicians' membership.

   Courtesy staff. This category includes health care providers qualified
for membership in the active organized staff who are permitted to admit
only a small number of patients each year to the facility. Courtesy staff
members are not eligible to vote or to hold office but are encouraged to
attend all meetings. Courtesy staff are usually on the active organized
staff of another hospital and often are held in higher professional regard
in their community.

   Consulting staff. The consulting organized staff consists of health care
providers who act only as consultants in their fields of specialty. They do
not vote or hold office in the organized staff but may attend all staff meetings and may be asked to serve on committees.

   Honorary staff. This category consists of health care providers who
are not necessarily active in the hospital and whom the hospital wishes
to honor as delineated in the hospital bylaws.

   Affiliate staff. The affiliate staff consists of allied health professional
and ancillary or paramedical personnel who have been granted limited
privileges by the organized staff to participate in patient care under the
direct and continued supervision of a member of the active or courtesy
organized staff. Affiliate staff usually do not have voting privileges and do
not serve on committees of the organized staff. They may be required to
attend and participate in the organized staff meetings. Historically, psychologists have been able to obtain privileges without benefit of state law
only as affiliate staff.
   Although the categories of organized staff describe the general privileges and responsibilities of health care providers, they do not indicate the
specific roles, functions, and limits of practice for individual staff members.
These specific practice limitations are called *privileges*, and the process of
gaining these privileges is described next.

Application for Staff Membership and Clinical Privileges

Application Process

Medical/professional staff membership and clinical privileges may be extended to applicants on the basis of the staff bylaws. In particular, the

sections about membership, credentials, review, and allied health personnel or affiliates to medical staff contain information about such issues as membership access, privileges, credential review, and medical supervision. With this information, psychologists can determine their level of eligibility for staff membership and privileges.

Each applicant is evaluated on an individual basis. Formal application is made to the medical staff, reviewed by the credentials committee, and recommended to the executive committee of the medical staff. The credentials committee is composed of health care providers who evaluate applications and make recommendations for staff status to the governing board.

Delineation of Privileges

Although laws and regulations may vary from state to state, a variety of privileges may be granted to psychologists. (See Exhibit 3.2 for a listing of privileges and roles that psychologists perform in a hospital setting.) These roles and privileges are currently being performed by psychologists with appropriate training and experience. The list is meant to be illustrative rather than exhaustive, as privilege decisions are based on the qualifications of individuals, and individual psychologists are qualified to provide a wide range of services. Psychologists should endeavor to gain explicit approval for the services they provide rather than permitting the institution to allow them to function in an informal fashion. Appendix A contains sample forms that psychologists may use to help them organize their application for privileges.

Renewal of Clinical Privileges

Renewal of clinical privileges is based on reappraisal of the individual at the time of reappointment. The results of quality assurance activities and other reasonable indicators of continuing qualifications, as well as peer and departmental recommendations, are included in the reappraisal. Participation in continuing education activities that relate to the privileges granted may also be considered.

Participation in Medical Staff Governance

As members of an independent autonomous profession, psychologists should participate in self-governance responsibilities and should be voting members of the medical staff. Within the organizational structure of a particular institution, psychologists should participate in the hospital and in the department or clinical service processes that have the responsibility for delineating privileges, reviewing credentials, and renewing privileges. The specific mechanism that is used to involve the psychologists will necessarily vary from one hospital to another. What is essential is that psychologists actively participate with their colleagues from medicine and other disciplines in these processes.

Exhibit 3.2.   Possible Hospital Privileges for Psychologists

Clinical Attending Privileges

Patient Management Privileges
- admit patients
- discharge patients
- coordinate and provide psychological care
- write and sign treatment plans
- write orders for assessment and treatment procedures
- write orders for medical, consultation, and other nonmedical services as needed
- supervise staff and trainees
- enter consultation notes on charts
- other, as appropriate

Clinical Assessment Privileges
- behavioral assessment
- biobehavioral and psychophysiological assessment
- neuropsychological examination
- mental status examination
- intellectual assessment
- personality assessment
- forensic assessment
- vocational/educational assessment
- psychosocial assessment
- other, as appropriate

Clinical Treatment Privileges
- individual psychotherapy
- group psychotherapy
- family psychotherapy
- behavior modification
- hypnosis
- biofeedback
- emergency room care/crisis intervention
- pain management
- rehabilitation services
- other, as appropriate

Consulting Privileges
- consultation liaison to other services, as needed
- organizational development services within the facility
- professional and community education
- staff development
- program planning and evaluation

Scientific Activities
- design scientific and clinical research, including individual case studies, control group studies, and program evaluation
- direct conduct on above research

Appealing Denial of Staff Membership or Privileges

In implementing staff membership and privileging procedures, each facility and agency should formulate and apply reasonable, nondiscriminatory standards for evaluating an applicant's credentials. As part of its overall responsibility for the operation of a facility or agency, the governing body, or people so designated, should ensure that decisions on clinical privileges and staff membership are based on an objective evaluation of an applicant's credentials, free of anticompetitive intent or purpose. Whenever possible, the credentials committee and other staff who evaluate the qualifications of applicants for clinical privileges and staff membership should include members of the applicants' profession.

Psychologists should be aware that their applications for membership and privileges may be turned down for a variety of reasons. The rationale for such denials should be available in writing and should be based on factors related to a psychologist's knowledge, experience, and demonstrated competence. If any of the following factors are considered in determining a psychologist's qualification for staff membership or clinical privileges, or if they play a part in denying a psychologist's privileges, the psychologist should appeal the decision and consider such other administrative and legal steps as are appropriate:

- an applicant's membership or lack of membership in a professional society or association;
- an applicant's decision to advertise, lower fees, or engage in other competitive acts intended to solicit business;
- an applicant's participation in prepaid group health plans, salaried employment, or any other manner of delivering health services on other than a fee-for-service basis;
- an applicant's support for, training of, or participation in a private group practice with members of a particular class of health professionals;
- an applicant's practices with respect to testifying in malpractice suits, disciplinary actions, or any other type of proceeding;
- an applicant's willingness to send a certain number of patients or clients to a particular hospital.

Each hospital should have procedures formulated to ensure that the foregoing factors play no part when decisions regarding clinical privileges and staff membership are made. The professional staff bylaws should provide the applicant with explicit procedures to be followed in instituting an appeals process if membership or privileges are denied (see Exhibit 3.3). It may be helpful to have the appeals process reviewed by an attorney and the state psychological association to make sure that the process meets statutory requirements and does not discriminate against psychologists as a class.

If the denial is based on a state regulation or statute that prohibits membership of psychologists or other factors beyond the control of the

Exhibit 3.3. Model Language That Can Be Used in Hospital Medical
Staff Bylaws

---

1. Medical staff: The categories of the medical staff must be defined. The medical
    staff will consist of active, consulting, and so forth.
2. Active medical staff: The prerogatives and criteria must be defined. The active
    medical staff will comprise physicians, dentists, and psychologists (or other
    health care practitioners) who have a currently valid and unrestricted license
    to practice in the state of _____. Only members of
    the active medical staff will be eligible to vote or hold office. All members of
    the active medical staff will have [specify category] clinical privileges.
3. Consulting medical staff: The consulting medical staff will consist of physicians,
    dentists, and psychologists (or other doctoral-level health care practitioners)
    who have a currently valid and unrestricted license to practice in the state of
    _____. Members of the consulting medical staff will
    have [specify category] privileges. They will not be able to hold office or to vote.
4. Clinical privileges: The delineation of clinical privileges needs to address pa-
    tient management functions and responsibilities such as the admission and
    discharging of patients and order writing. The delineation of privileges also
    needs to address health care services and responsibilities. For psychologists,
    this will mean the provision of psychological services. Moreover, psychological
    services will need to be defined. This can be accomplished by formulating a
    definition that includes the functions of assessment, consultation, diagnosis,
    and treatment. If the state law includes a definition of psychological services,
    that definition could be adopted.

---

hospital, it is likely the denial cannot be appealed on an individual basis.
Legislative change or litigation is probably indicated, and support from
local, state, and national professional organizations must be sought.

Sanctioning Psychologist Members

Finally, the role of psychologists on the medical staff includes participation
in the development of policies and procedures for sanctioning psychologist
members of the medical staff who do not follow the medical staff rules and
regulations or bylaws. Criteria for imposing sanctions should be consistent
with policy as found in the APA "Ethical Principles" (APA, 1992) and APA
"General Guidelines" (APA, 1987). Due process must be ensured, and all
procedures must conform with written hospital policy, medical staff bylaws, and the applicable state and federal statutes.

4 _____

The Culture of the Hospital: Rules and Procedures for Survival in a Hospital Practice

As psychologists move to expand their practices to include functioning in hospitals and other organized health facilities, it is important for them to understand the relationships that they will develop with and in these organizations. Psychology has worked for many decades to achieve legal recognition of the profession as an autonomous discipline with all of the rights, duties, and responsibilities of other professions. The field has been successful in this endeavor because psychology is a publicly regulated profession in all of the legal jurisdictions in the United States. APA ethics, standards, and guidelines, along with federal and state laws and regulations, provide the foundation on which the practice of psychology is based. As the autonomous status of the discipline has grown, psychologists increasingly have become accustomed to making decisions and taking responsibility for the services that they provide.

The status of all independent practitioners is clouded immediately when they move into organized settings to provide services. This is particularly true for psychologists who seek privileges to practice in hospitals. Although it remains true that the psychologists in a hospital setting continue to be recognized legally as autonomous professionals, the mere act of affiliating with an institution that is based on a complex multidisciplinary approach to patient care forces any health care provider to become dependent on the expertise and performance of other professions. The recognition of this interdependency represents a large step in psychologists' being able to function effectively in hospitals. It is important to note that permission granted by state licensing laws to use any particular treatment, for example, hypnosis, biofeedback, and even psychotherapy, is subject to some limitations when practitioners agree to abide by the hospital's bylaws.

In addition, psychologists must realize that hospitals have evolved their methods of operation over a long period of time in response to a unique set of environmental demands. Many of the rules and procedures are in place because of legal and regulatory requirements. They represent institutions' efforts to adapt to the constraints of their external and internal environments. To be sure, psychologists must remain vigilant regarding inappropriate or gratuitous procedures that undercut their autonomy. The most critical factor, however, is that psychologists must learn how to function within these organizations and to use the knowledge and resources of the other professionals and the organizations themselves if psychologists are to further their own development and to meet the needs of patients.

Medical Concerns for the Psychologist

What follows is a summary of some of the major issues and procedures that psychologists should understand as they begin to work in hospitals.

The reason for admitting a patient to a hospital generally revolves around either medication or physical concerns that need to be addressed and either cannot be done on an outpatient basis or must be performed specifically in a hospital setting. Either intensity of service or severity of illness criteria must be met to document the need for hospitalization. In most institutions where psychologists have privileges, it is the responsibility of the psychologist to arrange for the participation of a physician in matters of a medical nature. That involvement generally will include responsibility for physical health care, including medical examinations, prescribing and monitoring medications when appropriate, and neurological examinations where appropriate. Ideally, a psychologist will work in tandem with a physician to provide psychological input to the medical process and outcome, assuring high-quality, holistic care for the patient.

Usually, when a patient is admitted to a hospital, state law or a medical staff bylaw requires a medical examination to be completed within a certain number of hours of admission to the hospital. This examination provides a medical review of physical factors that might contribute to a patient's emotional difficulties. A psychologist, therefore, needs to develop a strong working relationship with a physician in order to evaluate quickly and effectively what a patient needs. Depending on how the hospital defines *medical exams*, it may or may not be appropriate for a psychologist to write orders for such things as specialty medical consultations, computerized tomography (CT) scans, or other laboratory procedures.

Physical exams and neurological exams may be essential for the appropriate treatment of a patient and, therefore, should be carried out quickly. The results of the exams should be communicated to the psychologist, and he or she should be intimately familiar with these results, in order to direct more appropriately the treatment of his or her patient. When medications are in order, the psychologist consults with a physician, to be well informed about the side effects that specific medications can cause. Communication by the patient of any side effects should be quickly brought to the attention of the physician, so that appropriate changes in the medications can be made. In addition, the psychologist is qualified to contribute scientifically based evaluations of behavior change due to drug administration. Communication between psychologists and physicians should therefore be a two-way process.

With the improvements made in biochemical assays and analysis, there is much that can be done these days to test for blood levels of certain medications to make sure that they are at a level that is therapeutic for the patient. Psychologists should be familiar with these procedures and with the availabilities of these tests. Side effects of psychotropic medications can often be very frightening and sometimes hazardous to the health of the patient. Side effects such as akathisia, Parkinsonian side effects, tardive dyskinesia, sexual dysfunction, dry mouth, and blurry vision should all be familiar to psychologists, so that they can be communicated to the physician should the patient complain of them.

Laboratory tests are often ordered while the patient is in the hospital. It would behoove psychologists to be able to converse in the language of the physician about lab tests and their importance to their patients. Lab tests include a number of different types of blood tests, urinalyses, and tests of levels of medications in the blood. Other more popular tests, such as electroencephalograms (EEGs), electrocardiograms (EKGs), CT scans, and X-rays, should also be familiar to psychologists. Psychologists should not attempt to interpret any of these medical tests, however, but should seek the counsel of the physician. Conversely, psychologists may be able to provide crucial neuropsychological data to be considered in conjunction with strictly medical data.

Medical emergencies are another area of concern. These may result from many different circumstances, such as from medication or changes in medication, from heart attacks, or from psychosomatic symptoms secondary to psychotherapeutic confrontations. Additionally, it may be appropriate for a patient to be maintained in seclusion or in restraints. All these considerations should be understood by psychologists before they ever work with a patient in a hospital. Should seclusion or restraint be necessary, psychologists should understand whether they are privileged to write orders for such and, if so, how these orders are written. Psychologists must also be aware of legal mandates and the individual hospital's policy regarding the restriction of patients' civil rights.

Treatment-Team Meetings

Many psychiatric hospitals and psychiatric units of general hospitals use a treatment-team approach. As such, there are a number of individuals who interact with the patient on a day-to-day basis. Although a psychologist may have admitted the patient to the hospital, the reality is that the admitting professional may deal with that patient only 3 to 6 hours a week during the patient's stay in the hospital. The other staff must deal with the patient on a day-to-day basis. Staff will often meet in what are called *treatment-team meetings* to define how the patient should be treated and what approach should be taken to treatment. It is at this point that orders written by the psychologist and other professionals are reviewed and that the implementation of these orders is discussed. Team meetings provide an important opportunity for psychologists to clarify their role.

It may also be a requirement when treating a patient in the hospital that the psychologist attend a treatment-team meeting to promote continuity of care to the patient. The treatment team basically discusses the patient's day-to-day activities. Often this is the only time that many of the different treating professionals from different disciplines get together to talk about a patient. It enables convergence of data on the patient's activities that allows the treatment plan to be updated on an appropriate basis. It also allows for the integration of plans from different disciplines to dovetail with each other, so that people are not working at odds with each other. Treatment-team meetings are a time for clarifying those orders that might be misunderstood and miscommunicated. They allow the psychologist an opportunity to learn what is happening with his or her patient.

A caution to psychologists going to team meetings: The team always has a full schedule. Your patient is not the only one being discussed at that time. Remember not to take too long in talking about your patient with the treatment team. Try to keep your focus on the goals for treatment of the patient, answering any questions that the treatment team has but not using up all of the team's limited time on your particular patient.

On-Call Requirements

As part of the professional staff of a hospital, psychologists may be required to be on call. This may mean accepting calls for certain periods of time, or it may mean being required to be in the hospital. On-call status should be clarified with the hospital at the time privileges are requested. Being on call is a major responsibility, and people depend on psychologists to respond to calls when they are made. The on-call status of psychologists is basically backup to the treating staff; it allows the treating staff to feel secure in what they are doing. It also allows the treating staff to define what changes in treatment should be made immediately in response to changes in a patient's behavior or condition.

Billing

In providing services to patients in a hospital setting, the issue of billing reimbursement should be clarified with the hospital, patients, and other responsible parties. Given the marked ongoing changes in hospital financing and reimbursement methodologies, it is incumbent upon psychologists to become conversant with the complex issues and procedures in this area. These issues include, but are not limited to, diagnosis-related groupings (DRGs), other forms of prospective reimbursement, fee schedules, and other special insurance reimbursement mechanisms such as those for preferred provider organizations (PPOs) and health maintenance organizations (HMOs). In collecting fees from insurance companies for services rendered, adherence to the documentation requirements is critical. The following sections describe these requirements.

Documentation Requirements

Hospitals must follow numerous and often conflicting regulations about the treatment of their patients. Because of this, psychologists may be required to document everything they do in a hospital. Psychologists must be prepared to do this in a form that is appropriate to the hospital. Depending on the hospital, documentation may need to be done in the problem-oriented medical records format or in another format designated by the hospital. Psychologists should be familiar with documentation formats before admitting a patient or attempting to write in a patient's chart. Documentation requirements for psychologists may include all of the following and more: admitting notes, consultation notes, treatment plans, psychological testing reports, progress notes, orders that are written on the chart, and discharge summaries.

Admitting Notes

An admitting note is a document written at the time of admission, so that the staff who will be working directly with the patient has an idea of what to do with that patient. The admitting note gives the staff a great amount of information that they must have in order to treat the patient appropriately. It is important that the note be written in a clear manner and in language that is easy to understand by all staff concerned. Staff who will be working with the patient includes highly trained nurses and minimally skilled aides, who must interpret what the psychologist wants done with that particular patient. The treatment team may have little knowledge of psychological terminology, so psychologists must use commonly understood language. An admitting note may contain all or part of the following:

Preliminary diagnosis. The preliminary diagnosis is important for many reasons. Patients must have a diagnosis for both treatment and regulatory reasons. It is therefore important that psychologists be familiar with *ICD–10* Diagnostic and Procedure Codes and the *Diagnostic and Statistical Manual of Mental Disorders*, 4th ed. (*DSM–IV*; American Psychiatric Association, 1994) and use these diagnostic nomenclatures as appropriate.

History of the current problem. The history should indicate why the patient is being hospitalized instead of being treated outside the hospital. Significant information may be given about the current event and current life situation that have made it difficult for the patient to cope on the outside.

Past treatment. The admitting note should also include documentation of treatment that the patient has received previously. It may be important to state if the patient has ever been hospitalized or treated for psychiatric or physical illness. If these factors are known, the response to various treatments should be documented, so that these treatments can either be ruled out or attempted fairly quickly on admission.

Current medications. Psychologists should describe medications that the patient is known to be taking, including the brand names, the ailments for which medications have been prescribed, and the dosages in which the medications have been taken. Psychologists should note past medications that the patient has been on, whether the patient is currently on them, and any reasons for discontinuing that medication in the past.

Physical problems and disorders. It is also generally helpful if psychologists can identify the problems and disorders that the patient may have concurrent but not necessarily associated with the mental or emotional problem.

Mental status exams. A mental status exam, which gives the treatment staff an indication of how the patient can be approached and what the patient can be expected to understand about his or her hospitalization, should be performed. The exam also gives the staff some indication of how cooperative the patient will be and what the patient's feelings are toward hospitalization. It should also suggest how the patient perceives reality, how the patient conceptualizes events, what the patient's current relationships are, and how appropriately the patient can express emotions that may be experienced.

In conjunction with the mental status exam, staff members should be given explicit instructions on how to approach the patient and how to deal with the patient while they are on the ward. This should include any particular situations that may result in the patient losing control or wanting to sign out against medical advice from the hospital.

Special precautions. Special precautions should be considered carefully with each patient. All patients should be asked, for example, whether they have any allergies. Although patients will be asked this question by other professionals in the hospital, it is helpful if the treating psychologist also asks and puts it in the admitting note. Other special precautions may include forensic involvement, suicidal tendencies, and so forth.

Initial Treatment Plan

The hospital may request a treatment plan subsequent to the admitting note. This treatment plan helps to guide both the psychologist and other treating staff toward the goals that the patient needs to reach during hospitalization. The hospital may or may not have a specific treatment plan form, but each treatment plan requires specific types of information, which fall into general categories. First, all requests for medical workup, including a physical examination, should be noted in the initial treatment plan. Although this will probably be taken care of automatically, it is appropriate to request it in writing. It often is said in hospital settings, "If it wasn't written down, it wasn't done." This must be understood very clearly by psychologists as a mandate for documenting all things that they request and that they do with the patient. The next thing that psychologists must take into account is what hospital services to offer the patient. These services may include activity therapy, social services, the services of a religious counselor, and other services that the patient may need while in the hospital.

In developing the initial treatment plan, it is essential that psychologists get recommendations from the treatment team about how to approach the patient. This encourages the team's interaction in developing a concerted effort toward treating a patient in the shortest time possible. It is important to know what expertise team members have (and to let them know what your expertise is), how they can help this patient, and how that fits into the overall treatment plan. Of course, the patient must be involved in his or her own treatment planning to the fullest extent possible. All voluntary treatment proceeds only on the basis of informed consent.

In many psychiatric settings, there is a classification or category system for the patient, which allows him or her more or less freedom within the hospital and is based on an assessment of the patient's control of his or her behavior, thinking, and perception. Categories may also regulate the number of visitors that a patient can have during hospitalization. This should be explained thoroughly to the patient, as well as to family members, and should be specified in the initial treatment plan. The two areas of greatest importance within the initial treatment plan are the short- and long-term goals.

Short-term goals. Short-term goals are those that can be accomplished within a short time and should be specific and defined so that the patient and the treatment team know what goals need to be accomplished. These should be specific behavioral accomplishments that can be observed, charted, and documented.

Long-term goals. Long-term goals should be identified for the patient as those that can be accomplished during the full length of hospitalization or following discharge. These may be the same as the short-term goals or they may be different, depending on how long the patient is going to be in the hospital, resources available after discharge, and so forth. These goals should specify those changes that must be accomplished before the patient is able to resume a normal life once outside the hospital setting.

Progress Notes

The progress note documents all things that are done with the patient. A progress note should include the following: (a) the date and time of the service; (b) the length of the service, such as an individual session for 30, 60, or 120 minutes; (c) the type of service, such as individual psychotherapy, group psychotherapy, and diagnostic testing; and (d) the name and degree or title of the individual rendering the service.

The progress note should relate to the original treatment plan or an updated treatment plan, identifying what the practitioner is doing with that patient and how that relates to the particular goals that were set. Progress notes also should be timely. A note that appears on the chart 1 week after the visit to the patient is essentially useless to the treating staff that is there with the patient 24 hours a day. A progress note, therefore, should be on the chart as immediately after rendering the service as possible. Although a progress note does not have to be lengthy, it should describe in succinct, understandable, and legible language what was done with the patient, how the patient responded, and what concerns either the psychologist or treating staff should have about the patient's response.

Progress notes are important for several reasons. JCAHO requirements are stringent about documenting what is done with a patient. These requirements are surveyed frequently in the hospital setting by both peer-review and quality-assurance meetings, to check on the quality, accuracy, and timeliness of the notes. These notes are also helpful in the legal sense in that they protect both the patient and the psychologist by documenting what services have been rendered and what the type of service was.

Progress notes are particularly important to the medical records department, which is charged with maintaining the records of the patients and assuring that those records are kept in good form. Progress notes also document information for billing and allow third-party payers to confirm when and what services were rendered.

Behavioral Orders

Psychologists with privileges in a hospital should be able to write orders on the patient's chart. These orders, however, will be limited according to the psychologist's privileges within the hospital. Examples of behavioral orders include some of the following, usually given in the course of inpatient treatment on a psychiatric unit.

Patient category or status. A patient on an inpatient psychiatric unit is assigned a category or classification of status, which tells other hospital staff how much independence or freedom a patient can have in his or her daily activities. These categories often define whether patients will be on a locked or open unit, able to leave the treatment unit, and able to attend certain types of therapeutic activities. They may also define certain privileges that patients may or may not have, such as the ability to have cigarettes and smoke by themselves, the ability to go to a day room or group room, or other such activities.

Visitation. If patients are in a psychiatric unit in the hospital, it is often because they cannot tolerate their lives outside the hospital, which includes family and friends. The psychologist should write orders as to who may visit, how often they may visit, and other visiting privileges that the patients may have. It should always be kept in mind that visiting privileges, except in very special circumstances, must be in line with the visiting policy of the hospital.

Passes. Giving therapeutic passes to patients for time away from an inpatient unit is often necessary. It may be important for a patient to practice relating to family, friends, or an employer before being discharged from the hospital. Psychologists take legal responsibility for the actions of a patient while he or she is on the pass. Thus, the psychologist defines the emotional stability of the patient and the ability of that patient to operate independently, keeping in mind both the welfare of the patient and that of others.

Activities. All other types of group, individual, or unit activities should be documented as an order. Otherwise a patient may not be permitted to participate in those activities.

Interventions. If it is appropriate to the psychologist's privileges, he or she may have the responsibility of writing seclusion or restraint orders, which are very closely monitored by the hospital. Again, state laws and hospital rules should be checked by psychologists before ordering such interventions, because these activities are often legally regulated. In addition, hospitals often have a special behavior-management or other such committee to monitor and review treatment procedures that restrict patients' civil rights.

Behavioral treatment. In many hospitals, psychologists are the only professionals allowed and expected to write time-out and other behavioral treatment orders. Such orders must be clearly communicated, properly implemented, and evaluated if they are to be effective. Psychologists must be aware of whatever legal restrictions relevant to the behavioral treatments exist.

Discharge summaries. Psychologists will probably be required to write for each patient a discharge summary, which is a formal document specifying what treatment the patient has received during the time in the hospital. It is this document that is often sent out to other professionals when they request information on the patient's hospitalization. There are a number of things that this document should contain:

- Course in the hospital: Essentially, documentation of a patient's course should explain how a patient accepted treatment at first, progressed through treatment, and responded to the treatment and his or her status at time of discharge.
- Procedures, tests, or medicines: Any procedures, tests, or medicines that were administered to the patient during the course of treatment in the hospital should be documented and a summary of those results given.
- Critical incidents: Any critical incidents that occurred during a patient's hospitalization that changed the course of treatment of the patient, changed the patient's outlook on the treatment, or required special procedures on the part of the treating staff should be described in the discharge summary.
- Discharge follow-up: Follow-up should specify what treatment will be given subsequent to hospitalization and where and by whom the treatment will be offered.
- Discharge diagnosis: If the discharge diagnosis is different from the admitting diagnosis, clarification of the reasons for the change should be documented.

Some General Suggestions for Psychologists Working in Hospitals

The following are commonsense tips to facilitate relationships in the hospital setting.

Use English, Not "Psychologese"

Reports and consultations are not being written, for the most part, for other mental health care providers. They characteristically are being written for others on the treatment team—registered nurses (RNs), licensed practical nurses (LPNs), medical doctors (MDs), and others. Make sense; avoid using psychological terminology that will not be understood by nonpsychologists. For example, do not say, "Patient overuses defense mechanisms of repression and denial." Say instead, "Patient doesn't want to admit this to himself." Say, "Patient should be encouraged to be more active, both socially and physically" rather than "Patient has decathected." Distinguish clearly between your perceptions and learned interpretation of the patient's behaviors, for example, "The patient struck a nurse in the head, apparently out of anger toward her limit setting."

Be Action Oriented

Hospitals are intervention-oriented institutions. They do things to people, and generally the staff and treatment team want to know what to do. It is generally not helpful in establishing rapport with staff and other providers to talk only about insight and feelings in response to their questions. If staff members ask what to do, tell them. Generally, when it comes to matters of behavior and emotional treatment, you are seen as the pilot of a plane. To abdicate this role may increase the passengers' anxiety.

Be Brief

Consultation reports of more than one page generally will not be read by many medical specialists. Rather than impressing them with your thoroughness, you would be impressing them negatively with your inconsideration for their time, with your inability to be succinct and to the point, and with your lack of knowledge of how hospitals function.

Know What You Are Doing and Know Your Limits

If you do not know specific information about medicines for psychosis, anxiety, and affective disorders, do not bluff. If you do not know about side effects of medicines prescribed for physical problems, sequelae to certain treatments, or course and aftermath of certain conditions, ask or say that you do not know. Once credibility is lost, it is difficult to regain. Most medical practitioners realize that they do not know all answers to all questions and do not expect others to know all the answers, either. Learn the language, acronyms, and abbreviations used in charts before you use them.

Be Polite, Friendly, and Helpful When It Is Appropriate

Your first time on a ward, determine who the charge nurse is and introduce yourself. Talk with nurses, make friends with ward secretaries, acknowledge helpful nurses' notes or actions, and give encouraging and honest reactions to others on the treatment team. Learn names and use them. The best way to assure cooperation with your treatment plan is to demonstrate that you can carry it out with your patient, for example, by setting limits with intimidating or assaultive patients and by teaching social skills.

Let the Self-Fulfilling Prophecy Work for You

Do not anticipate rejection. You are not a second-class citizen but will be welcomed by most of the hospital staff and personnel as a valuable member of the treatment team. Do not view yourself as a guest in someone else's house. You have a right to be there so long as your goal is to contribute to the care of patients. Do not anticipate an adversarial relationship with anyone, but remember that the laws of society and principles of economics, as well as people's general desire for peaceful affiliation, will ultimately validate your role and overcome initial conflicts or coolness. Mutual respect of competencies is crucial to interdisciplinary team functioning.

Be Sensitive to the Need for Flexibility in How You Practice

There is much variation among how a surgical ward, a pediatric unit, an emergency room, and an inpatient mental health unit operate. Respond to what is appropriate to the context you are in.

Do Not Form Alliances on the Treatment Team

From time to time one might see some conflicts between various people or factions in hospitals. Do not try to patch these up unless your role is that of organizational consultant. If your role is taking care of a patient, do this and ignore staff problems unless problems interfere with patient care. If necessary, particularly if a conflict affects patient care, use the established hierarchy of the hospital to resolve such conflicts.

Respect the Hierarchy of the Institution

It might be less than effective on a medical ward to explain things to an LPN and to avoid telling things to the RN, who outranks the LPN. Roles and role relationships are important in hospital settings.

Part II

Advocacy Issues in Hospital Practice

5

Strategies for Acquiring Medical Staff Membership

In this chapter and the next, we turn to two particular areas related to hospital practice. This chapter deals with strategies for acquiring medical staff membership in a specific hospital; chapter 6 focuses on enacting state legislation and federal agency rule changes to enable independent practice for psychologists in hospitals.

Participation in hospital services immediately involves the professional in multidisciplinary professional services and relations, an environment that is far less insular than office-based practice. These new contacts can be avenues for expanded professional opportunity. Some of the hospitals will become highly successful as community treatment centers with a network of outpatient services, satellite clinics, professional office centers, and continuing educational conferences. They will become a nucleus of community health activities, whether they are free-standing, linked with a chain of hospitals, or part of an HMO system like Kaiser Permanente.

It is important, therefore, to gain medical staff standing at a viable hospital. It will be a major plus for both professional development and the range of professional activities. It will also help to offset the negative impact of a shrinking independent private-office practice due to the progressive penetration of managed care organizations (MCOs) into the health care marketplace. Also, medical-staff membership in a hospital or formal standing to practice in another type of hospital can facilitate the acquisition of contracts with MCOs, which prefer providers who can render services in a range of settings and which increasingly need to assure a sufficient provider-to-enrollee ratio to assure access to quality care.

Not just hospitals, but all health care facilities, public or private, will have a medical or professional staff organization. Such organizations are demanded by the federal government of any facility receiving Medicare or Medicaid funds. They are demanded by accrediting bodies such as JCAHO and are typically demanded by state licensing agencies. The organizations are there, and this book is intended to provide background facts to assist psychologists in their efforts to acquire staff status in hospitals.

Psychologists who specialize in health care services and have professional experience in licensed hospitals are more than likely qualified applicants for medical staff membership. Psychological health services are provided in psychiatric hospitals (public and private); psychiatric units of acute general medical hospitals, including structured outpatient services; medical and surgical units of general hospitals; university hospitals; nursing homes; rehabilitation centers; hospices; substance-abuse treatment centers; day-treatment centers; counseling centers; HMOs; and industrial and school health clinics.

Practice patterns by psychologists within each of these settings will vary and, therefore, should be identified. The nature of the practice can best be classified according to (a) the range of services offered (narrow vs. broad privileges); (b) whether formally codified or agreed to verbally by local arrangement (formal vs. informal); (c) the basis for staffing (open vs. closed) and whether special criteria are used when psychologists apply for privileges (gender and ethnic diversity or specialist requirements, such as neuropsychology or child clinical, or staffing-to-bed-occupancy ratios); (d) the levels of staff membership open to psychologists (active, consulting, or affiliate staff); and (e) the extent of peer (psychologist) determination in the approval of new psychologist practice applications.

The roles they may assume can include providing clinical services, training personnel, directing group or family therapy programs, or designing and conducting clinical or outcome research. In addition to providing clinical services, psychologists may formulate treatment plans, write treatment orders, render diagnoses, conduct psychological assessment, supervise other therapists and trainees, or direct specific programs. Their skills and training qualify them to play an integral role in the hospital and the community that the hospital serves.

Community Resources

Psychologists interested in formally gaining practice privileges in a specific hospital, and willing to launch an effort to do so, must assess what resources are available to them in their community. This means they must identify individuals who can help them achieve their objective and then enlist the support and assistance of these individuals. Such an effort is time-consuming, but it must be done if psychologists are to gain privileges. First, local psychologists with an established hospital practice are among those resources that must be identified. Psychologists are encouraged to solicit their counsel and, if possible, develop a working, supportive relationship with them. Those established psychologists who already have expertise in coordinating and leading group efforts should be actively enlisted in the effort. Second, psychologists are urged to explore collaboration with other health care providers with similar goals. Third and most important, psychologists need to identify people in decision-making positions—such as hospital administrators, chief of the medical staff, specific department heads, and local political leaders—who can actually help determine the outcome of their advocacy effort. Without some external support, psychologists will find it difficult to secure the hospital privileges that they seek. And, of course, the credentials of the psychologist–

applicant are key. The sounder his or her hospital experience and the more contributions made to quality professional care, the more compelling the application.

Personal Contacts

As part of the effort to gain practice privileges in a hospital, psychologists should speak with several individuals and groups. These typically would include contacts at the hospital with leading psychologists in the community and with the executive officer of the state psychological association. Consultation with the APA's Practice Directorate office in Washington, DC, will also provide useful guidance.

The first approach to advocating for hospital medical staff membership is a personal one: people getting to know people. It is less difficult for a psychologist to seek membership if he or she knows a member of the medical staff (particularly the chief of the medical staff or the chair of the bylaws committee), the administrator, or an attorney of an institution. Making personal acquaintances and becoming familiar with the particular concerns of the hospital are essential steps in the advocacy process. Psychologists with a special expertise should offer to provide a continuing-education seminar or other presentation to facility staff.

In addition, established local psychologists should be approached. Some already have formal or informal relationships with hospitals or physicians to provide services, and many may work with patients with primarily physical problems. Thus, even though their practice may be primarily office based, they are not at risk of interrupting a patient's treatment if he or she needs hospitalization. These psychologists should be encouraged to use their personal contacts to assist the advocacy effort. Psychologists in group or corporate practice, particularly multidisciplinary groups and groups that have contracted to provide health or mental health services to people enrolled in a managed-care plan, will likely already have operational arrangements to admit and treat patients in contracting hospitals. They can be a valuable source of advice and professional contacts (see Exhibit 5.1).

Local Liaisons

In the advocacy effort, it is advantageous for psychologists to become acquainted with the hospital staff who are responsible for the day-to-day care and implementation of treatment plans, such as nurses and primary-care physicians who are directly and regularly involved in the main flow of patient services. They can be valuable allies. Physicians from whom you have received referrals or to whom you have made referrals should also be approached. In undertaking efforts to establish hospital staff membership, psychologists must assess their relationships with medical colleagues. Do physicians believe that having access to a psychologist with

Exhibit 5.1.   Checklist for Developing Community Resources

First, list the area's psychologists by name, address, and type and volume of their hospital practice.

Second, acquire names of all area institutions:
- hospitals, whether private, state, county, or district hospitals (including general, children's, psychiatric, and teaching);
- rehabilitation centers;
- community mental health centers with inpatient services;
- nursing homes and hospices;
- health maintenance organizations;
- independent practice associations and preferred provider organizations that contract to render local inpatient services and the facilities they use;
- managed care organizations (MCOs) that have contract agreements with local hospitals. Identify those MCO-contracted facilities and their psychologists (staff and network) with hospital privileges.

Third, evaluate current hospital practice patterns of area facilities. (How many have provided privileges to psychologists? What kind of privileges? How many employ psychologists as salaried staff?)

Fourth, identify and determine the individuals and resources that are or can be helpful:
- community resources (e.g., local psychologists with established hospital practices);
- community leaders, county supervisors;
- organizational contacts;
- local association strength;
- local experts, which may include not only clinical psychologists but also academicians, and locally respected physicians;
- sources of funding.

Fifth, develop a database.
- Secure a copy of the current edition of the JCAHO *Comprehensive Accreditation Manual for Hospitals* or, if more appropriate to the facility in question, the JCAHO *Manual for Mental Health, Chemical Dependency, and Mental Retardation/Developmental Disabilities Services.*
- Secure a copy of the specific hospital medical staff bylaws.
- Compare and evaluate these bylaws for compliance with state law and JCAHO accreditation standards.
- Evaluate all levels of hospital staff for their receptivity to including psychologists in their membership.
- Identify psychologists with and without privileges practicing in local facilities.
- Determine patient populations, licensed occupancy by target facility (this includes basic demographics: age and type of disorder), and average daily census.
- Review the annotated bibliography published in this volume for pertinent articles, and screen more recent publications for relevant articles.

---

your special expertise in the hospital is a benefit? Do they consider the psychologists' desire to secure hospital privileges to be an infringement on their medical practice? Do physicians anticipate a collegial relationship or a competitive one? This view may differ dramatically depending on the physician's specialty. The competitive reality that exists between psychiatry and psychology suggests that outright opposition can occur but does not have to. Other specialties—notably pediatricians, neurologists, internists, and family practitioners—are often very supportive of psychologists as clinical colleagues in hospitals.

The chief of the medical staff can be a powerful ally or adversary. It is important to meet this person and assess his or her attitude toward psychologists practicing in hospitals. Get to know those physicians who can provide positive support and can serve as advocates when approaching the medical director. The hospital administrator may also be an ally of psychologists. Usually more concerned with the administration of the facility and cash-flow revenue rather than professional turf battles, the administrator (who is often not a physician) may be more approachable and willing to advocate on behalf of psychology than the medical director.

It is incumbent on the psychologist seeking staff membership to determine first whether access to privileges is possible; the hospital with an *open* staff is where psychologists will want to first focus their attention because hospitals with a *closed* staff are usually staffed by invitation only. Moreover, the attitude or opportunity can differ significantly between hospitals in communities where there is more than one hospital. Once having gained membership in the organized staff, all practitioners are guided by hospital bylaws.

Local psychological associations can serve as catalysts to bring together various segments of the medical, hospital, political, and psychological communities for the purpose of exchanging information and perspectives and determining what resources are available. As a social organization, the local association can sponsor professional and community events, with featured speakers from the hospital and the local member of the state legislature or officers of city or county government, or develop alliances with members of other concerned professions.

Local associations can provide a valuable function for both the psychologists and the hospital by serving as a practice-standards review committee. The JCAHO requires that practitioners applying for staff membership be able to demonstrate that they are in good standing with the profession and the community. The local association can supply such confirmation, usually in writing, in a manner acceptable to both the psychologist and the hospital. The local association can also provide information on the suitability of the hospital-based practice of psychologists and on the appropriateness of the training of psychologists who apply for membership.

Psychologists also should use the valuable public relations and marketing services that local associations can offer. These associations can help convey to hospitals the monetary benefits of granting hospital privileges to psychologists, which is important in times when hospitals are looking for ways to improve fiscal performance and expand their purview. One such benefit is the direct impact psychologists can have on census (patient admissions) by admitting their patients to the institution. Another benefit is that in addition to providing specialized behavioral health care, psychologists can supply professional expertise in other areas of health care, including pediatrics, internal medicine, neurology, surgery, and coronary care units. Psychological consultation also can help improve the overall quality of care and patients' compliance with medical advice. In short, psychological services should be attractive to any hospital interested in enhancing its efficiency and the effectiveness of their health care system.

In states where legislation or regulations have been implemented recognizing hospital practice by psychologists, the state psychological association can be a particularly valuable resource. As of 1998, there were 17 such states or districts.[3] Not only can the state psychological associations in these jurisdictions inform specific hospitals of the law but they are also in a position to provide support to their members seeking membership in the facility staff. In addition to these states with a specific law or regulation enabling the hospital practice of psychology, there are 15 other states where the laws are silent or generic with terms such as *licensed professional* or *hospital staff member*. These states include Alaska, Arizona, Idaho, Massachusetts, Michigan, Minnesota, Nebraska, New Hampshire, Oregon, Rhode Island, South Dakota, Virginia, Washington, West Virginia, and Wyoming. State psychological association support can certainly be helpful in these states as well. Indeed, with member interest in hospital practice, the association may be prompted to seek constructive legislation.

---

[3]See Appendix B for a listing of these states and the language of actual laws. The language is for illustrative purposes only. As state laws are subject to change, psychologists are advised to confirm the most current version. A legal analysis of existing hospital practice legislation is available from the APA Practice Directorate Legal and Regulatory Affairs Department.

6

Strategies for Legislative and Regulatory Changes

Psychologists and other health professions are licensed by the state. So are hospitals, health insurers, and health care service plans. Thus, every psychologist perforce must practice within state law or regulation whether in an office or hospital. Some federal laws, however, can override some aspects of state jurisdiction (e.g., the Health Maintenance Organization Development Act of 1973, among other things, negated state laws that disallowed the formation of HMOs and sought to preclude physicians from practicing in HMOs, and the Employee Retirement Income Security Act of 1974 (ERISA) exempted self-insured employers from state freedom-of-choice laws), and some federal health insurance laws (e.g., Medicare) have established conditions with which providers (professional and institutional) must comply in order to participate. If psychology wants to expand its scope of practice and have its services recognized and paid for, and does not want to be in conflict with the law, then psychology must change those laws that place unreasonable restraints on the practice of psychology or prevent a future expansion in scope of practice consistent with new developments in behavioral science. (For some background on legislative advocacy and illustration of specific law changes, see Bersoff, 1983; Dörken, 1981, 1983; Dörken & Carpenter, 1986; Dörken, VandenBos, Henke, Cummings, & Pallak, 1993; Reaves, 1984; and Tanney, 1985.)

Advocacy at the State Level

Changing state (or federal) law is most effectively and systematically accomplished by assembling the resources of one's professional association. Each state psychological association needs a legislative committee or office of governmental affairs to gain consensus on the priorities for change, the feasibility of change, the resources that will be required, and so on. State associations are well advised to work collaboratively with the APA Practice Directorate's Office of Legal and Regulatory Affairs and its Office of State Advocacy. With regard to hospital advocacy, even though a specific target, there are many aspects to consider.

Before launching an initiative to gain hospital staff membership legislation, state psychologists must first determine the provisions of their state codes on hospital organization. State laws may be silent, permissive, mandated, or prohibitive with respect to psychologists practicing in a hospital setting. Look also at other classes of health care facilities, such as rehabilitation centers, nursing facilities, developmental centers, and the several classes of public and private hospitals (both nonprofit and for profit). Also consider which services, if any, are required. To assist those seeking membership and privileges, the state association needs to conduct a thorough review of current laws and regulations regarding hospital credentialing. The psychology licensing act and mental health, commitment, and insurance laws need to be reconsidered in this context. These should be investigated, and corrective legislation should be developed to address both statutory and regulatory barriers to hospital practice.

Before legislation is developed, the state psychological association needs to be convinced of the necessity for legislative redress. This involves educating the board of directors as well as the membership at large. Psychologists need to become actively involved in the political process within their state and to establish themselves as politically influential. Each state association needs to have a lobbying organization to gain continuity of purpose. External lobbying costs for one specific piece of legislation can be expensive and may build no bridges. A political action committee (PAC) can also be formed to raise funds for political campaign contributions to candidates supportive of psychologists.

Although many psychologists react to the word *lobbying* as if it were anathema, it is essential to promote favorable legislation. Anything that is worth having is worth requesting. Lobbying is really nothing more than meeting and getting to know legislators, becoming familiar with issues of importance to them, and apprising them of psychology's interests and concerns and how psychology can contribute to improved health care. Any citizen may do this. The goal of lobbying is to inform legislators about a particular issue, seek a favorable hearing for legislation, and, where possible, gain a positive commitment from legislators for psychologists' interests regarding the issue.

To lobby effectively, psychologists should be aware of the legislative history regarding hospital privileges, what type of support or sponsorship the legislator can and will offer, what forces are or could be working against the legislation, what fiscal impact the legislation will have on state finances, how the legislation helps the constituents of the particular legislator or the people of the state in general, what specific law the legislation would change, whether the change might be part of a broader objective under consideration, such as revision of the mental health act, and when in the session it would come up for vote. The most important point of these concerns is the impact the legislation will have if it is enacted. The major underlying issue for psychology may be the profession's access to patients, whereas the opposition may be against such access and have cost and quality-of-care concerns. When psychologists provide data demonstrating the efficacy of hospital-based psychological practice, they underscore their need and their argument for hospital privileges. When presented positively, this information is critical to making a persuasive argument, and without it many legislators may remain unconvinced (Dörken, 1983). Another method of clarifying legislative intent is to ask a legislator for an attorney general's opinion to see whether a situation requires legislative redress. Although the opinion does not hold the force of law, it could help clarify issues and provide a sound argument for passage of the legislation.

It is important to know what implications a hospital-practice bill for psychologists will have for other statutes. For example, psychologists may wage a hard battle to have a hospital-practice bill passed only to find out that the state nursing practice act specifically prohibits nurses from taking orders from anyone other than a physician. This example illustrates the importance of doing thorough legislative research and knowing what other laws should be modified concurrently for a hospital practice bill to have maximum effect.

Organizations as Resources

Psychologists should encourage their state psychological associations to initiate and support efforts to obtain medical staff membership and independent practice privileges for psychologists in hospitals. This effort may take a substantial commitment of resources, possibly for several years.

If the state association is not currently involved in the issue of hospital practice, a standing or ad hoc committee should be established. Interest is fine, but experience is better. Some states may have more than one association, which may include, for example, an academy of practitioners. Such organizations can form alliances, pool resources, and provide a broader base of involvement and support. Such alliances could also include friendly organizations, such as those representing nurses, podiatrists, optometrists, or family practitioners.

Psychologists who work in a hospital may have formal or informal networks of communication that can be the nucleus of the advocacy group. These interpersonal networks may be able to work in conjunction with the state association to promote the advocacy effort. Similarly, local psychological associations are a potential resource. Most large cities and counties have a formal or informal organization of psychologists. Psychologists can coordinate state efforts to use all communication sources, including local groups, newsletters, journals, gatherings at state association meetings, and special local association meetings. It is of utmost importance that psychologists develop a broad, statewide support base if they are to effect change in hospital law as it will apply throughout the state. Because so many parties, professions, and economic interests are involved in legislation to change or expand who can practice in a hospital (and thereby change its licensing criteria), hospital-practice bills are some of the most difficult legislative proposals to pass. The real problem is not the effectiveness or quality of psychological services; the problem is public relational and political. There is a mass of culture, tradition, and public status quo acceptance that must be overcome or won over.

Political contacts are essential. It is much easier to convince a legislator who knows psychology to introduce and defend the legislation than to expect support from a legislator who has had no prior contact with the discipline. Passage is more likely if the author/legislator is a member of the legislative policy committee that will hear the bill.

Knowledgeable psychologists should make themselves available for the duration of the legislative session to monitor the bill's passage and assure that it receives attention in its progress through the legislature. These individuals need to be versed in the proposed legislation, the quality of psychological services, current law, potential opposition, and relevant psychological research. They must be able to advocate psychology's position and how it benefits the citizens of the state in a cost-effective manner.

Financial commitment by the state psychological association is essential to assuring competent legal assistance and effective communication with legislators. Telephone efforts, face-to-face visits with legislators, and the use of professional lobbyists are all proven methods of accomplishing these goals. As many of them as possible should be used.

Resources for Advocacy Efforts

Advocacy simply is pleading one's cause. It is an effort to secure what is wanted, which in this case is medical staff membership and privileges to practice in hospitals and other health care facilities (see Exhibit 6.1). To be effective, psychologists must acquire information in two areas: what constitutes a hospital practice and how psychologists can be participants. Part I of this book addresses issues relevant to hospital practice—for example, psychologists' roles and training, hospital organization, and bylaws. In contrast, this chapter addresses ways in which psychologists can engage hospitals politically and organizationally to obtain privileges. Although local situations may vary, the following facts apply nationally:

- Psychologists constitute the largest doctorally trained mental health profession. The number of psychologists now exceeds the number of psychiatrists in practice. By 1989, there were 56,530 doctoral-level licensed psychologists (Pion, Kohout, & VandenBos, 1990). According to APA, the number of doctoral-level licensed psychologists has grown to approximately 70,000 in 1998.
- To add a multidisciplinary perspective, the number of licensed psychologists is comparable to the number of optometrists, about six-fold greater than the number of nurse practitioners or podiatrists, about one ninth the number of physicians, and one fourth greater than the number of psychiatrists.
- Psychologists are licensed or certified for independent practice in all 50 states.
- Psychologists are recognized as independent providers in every fed-

Exhibit 6.1.   Checklist for Undertaking Advocacy Efforts

Appoint a separate hospital practice committee if one does not exist.

Assess current plans of the state psychological association for dealing with hospital practice issues.

Identify interested members of the state or local psychological association committed to the issue, particularly those who have membership/clinical privileges in a hospital setting.

Identify key members of the legislative committee who are friendly or need to be oriented.

Develop a network of psychologists who know or can contact state legislators.

Assess current state laws concerning the following:

- psychological licensing
- freedom of choice
- hospitals (public and private)
- medical practice act
- insurance
- nursing practice act
- nursing home licensing act
- rehabilitation facilities
- developmental centers
- correctional treatment centers

Assess potential support and opposition to changes in the law.

Identify local associations that will support and work actively in the effort.

Identify local hospital concerns and target hospital(s) and other hospitals.

Contact APA.

- Check files on state legislative activities.
- Inquire about contacts and established networks.
- Examine available research about current practice patterns.

Join advisory committees.

Join governmental planning groups; contact local liaisons.

Note. Everyone does not have to do everything. Depending on the state or community, some organizations will be far more pertinent than others. Be selective; focus on your target objective.

---

eral health care statute and insurance program and in the federal criminal code and the Federal Employees' Compensation Act (Workers' Compensation, 39 U.S.C. §742 [1916], as amended).

- Twenty-nine states have laws mandating or regulating minimum benefits or the availability of mental health services in insurance contracts. In some of these states, psychologists are specifically recognized in the state statutes. Furthermore, 42 states and the District of Columbia have enacted direct-recognition laws, commonly called *freedom of choice* (FOC), which assure third-party reimbursement for psychological services; 92% of the U.S. population (Dörken, Stapp, & VandenBos, 1986) reside in these states. (Self-insured employers, however, are exempted from state FOC laws under ERISA.)

- Sixty-one percent of all internships for psychologists in the United

States are in a hospital setting, such as Veterans Administration or teaching hospitals (Kurz, Fuchs, Dabek, Kurtz, & Helfrich, 1982).

- The JCAHO recognizes the legitimate claim of nonphysicians to hospital practice, to include membership on the medical staff of licensed health practitioners, and authorizes psychologists to write seclusion and restraint orders when permitted by state law and the facility.

The annotated bibliography in the back of this book also lists resources that may be useful in advocacy efforts.

Informing the state-association membership of the necessity of hospital-based practice through newsletters, special mailings, or convention programs is crucial. Support also can be garnered on a broad scale in the form of consciousness-raising on the part of all involved: psychologists, patients, legislators, physicians, hospital personnel, and the general public. However, the use of mass media, newspapers, and talk shows is best left for later, to report success and to then disseminate general public information and heighten awareness of the implications involved.

For these activities to be effective, fund-raising may have to be an integral part of the effort. The development of continuing education training programs that teach specific skills relative to practice in a hospital setting will help individual psychologists prepare for such practice. Additionally, some will need sites at which they can gain supervised clinical experience if that has not already been part of their professional preparation. Such programs also will help those who review credentials for the purpose of identifying qualified practitioners.

In some regions, groups of psychologists have formed coalitions that focus specifically on the hospital-practice issue. Contact with these groups can provide information about local hospital organizations and activities (e.g., regarding fiscal structure, membership, meeting frequency, or committee structure).

Organizations such as these have found that mailing a newsletter focusing on the hospital issue, with a tear-off sheet for readers to return to indicate interest, helps identify sources of support. Organizing conferences with speakers from APA or from states in which legislation has been passed can also crystallize issues and promote support. Furthermore, documents such as position papers or summaries of relevant laws and regulations can help educate those psychologists unfamiliar with the complexities of the issue, who could eventually be enlisted for support.

APA

APA has accumulated information on the issue of hospital practice for psychologists. The Practice Directorate maintains a current file on the legislative activities of most states. Staff can supply legislative or legal information regarding hospital-practice legislation, policy, litigation, and sample bylaws. They also can provide appropriate contacts with individuals in other states who are currently working on or have been successful in passing similar legislation. Additionally, the Directorate maintains files on research about the current practice patterns of psychologists, relevant national legislation and trends, and socioeconomic data on health care across the country.

APA can help psychologists establish networks and identify individuals who have been actively involved in securing hospital medical staff membership for psychologists. Close contact with APA's Practice Directorate can be beneficial. It is located at 750 First Street, NE, Washington, DC 20002-4242.

The Council for the National Register of Health Service Providers in Psychology

The Register not only is a credentialing service regarding a current and unrestricted license to practice but also verifies hospital staff membership. More than 2,000 psychologists are now listed. They can be a major resource.

Advisory Committees

Many states and localities have mental health or health care advisory committees that discuss relevant issues and offer recommendations to heads of government units, commissioners, legislators, and other public officials. Similarly, legislators themselves form study groups, task forces, and advisory committees on health care and related issues. Psychologists need to be represented in these groups. Obtaining membership on such a committee provides access to helpful individuals and to a wealth of useful information and provides a forum from which to influence health care policy decisions. Some committees are mandated by the governor, some by the legislature as study groups, and others are created by mental health associations, health departments, and so on. Within the state, psychologists need to be vigilant regarding the formation of such committees and then lobby to secure inclusion. It is far easier to gain constructive change as a member when change is under way than to try and change matters after the fact or to do so as an outsider.

Local government bodies or planning groups such as a Council of Government (COG) have health care components and often propose policies for local government consideration. Most states require long-term medical or mental health care plans, and having access to these plans and commenting on them are important. If possible, psychologists should seek to join these groups or their advisory bodies.

Coalitions

Coalitions are potentially powerful political forces when they address concerns such as state budgets, consumer issues, and patients' rights. Psychologists should join these groups to meet other providers on a personal level, to exchange information on health care, and to form alliances. Such alliances frequently are formed with other professionals (e.g., nurse practitioners and optometrists). Initial steps include conducting meetings with executive boards of these other professional groups on a state level, having lobbyists of the different groups confer, or inviting these groups to cosponsor a program at a state psychological association meeting. What is important is to make contact and begin to organize.

Finally, even though psychologists are reluctant to involve patients in issues other than treatment, there are precedents for such activity. Patients and their families vote in elections, and they can be regarded as potential allies in the fight for hospital privileges. Letters from patients to legislators will often provide more impetus to change than many hours of lobbying by psychologists. However, enlisting their support should be done with extreme caution because it could have negative implications for the therapeutic relationship and could be viewed as a conflict of interest for the therapist. It is sometimes easier to approach organized consumer groups, such as the state mental health association, conference of local mental health directors, and association for the mentally ill.

Components of a Suggested Hospital Practice Law

Note first that medical staff membership is the fundamental objective. It is from this that appropriate clinical privileges, plus committee memberships and the right to vote, flow. To open with a request for some specific privilege, such as the right to admit, can generate major local opposition, whereas seeking to provide only some clinical service, such as assessment or psychotherapy, is more in keeping with affiliate status, functioning on medical referral.

Here then are the desirable components of hospital-practice legislation:

1. The licensing law should clearly state that psychologists are licensed for independent practice, including the diagnosis and treatment of emotional, behavioral, and mental disorders and the psychological aspects of injury, disability, chronic disease, and dying. If not, that scope-of-practice issue may need prior resolution or inclusion in facility-practice legislation, perhaps with a more stringent definition of *clinical psychologist* or *health-service-provider psychologist*.
2. A health code or hospital licensing code should define the different types of hospital (e.g., general acute-care hospital or acute psychiatric hospital) and state the basic services that each provides. If services of physicians, nurses, and so forth are specified, then at some future time *psychologists* should be added. This guarantees that psychologists' professional services will become available but does not guarantee their membership on the medical staff.

3. The venue of psychologists to practice should be open in all manner of licensed health facilities, not simply hospitals or psychiatric hospitals.

4. There should be no prohibition or discrimination against licensed psychologists on the basis of their degree or license in employment, appointment to categories of the medical staff, or the granting of clinical privileges.

5. Depending on the situation, there should be penalties that can be imposed on a hospital that discriminates against licensed psychologists simply on the basis of their degree or license.

6. If a health service is offered by a hospital with both physicians and psychologists on staff and is one that both are authorized by law to perform, then it should be clear that the service can be provided by either without discrimination.

7. The bylaws of all licensed hospitals, public and private, should be required to establish provisions for the expeditious consideration of applications from qualified psychologists for medical staff membership or designated clinical privileges. Such applications should not be denied solely on the basis of licensure or degree.

8. The clinical privileges that may be granted to a psychologist should be within the licensed scope of practice and personal competence of the psychologist but may include and not be limited to diagnosis, treatment, treatment planning, psychological assessment and evaluation, record review, and the authorization to admit and discharge patients, any and all, without external direction or supervision by another professional.

9. Psychologists shall have peer representation in the selection of future psychologist applicants for medical staff membership and clinical privileges.

Federal Law

The Civilian Health and Medical Program of the Uniformed Services (CHAMPUS) has recognized psychologist inpatient services on a formal basis since 1977. In 1983, an annual 60-day limitation on inpatient mental health care was instituted (PL 97-377), but it provided an express waiver for "extraordinary medical or psychological circumstances," clearly underscoring that the recognition of psychological services included in-patient care. This cap was reduced to 30 days, effective April 1992. Additionally, the Federal Employee Health Benefit Plan has not discriminated against psychologist inpatient services since 1974, when it recognized clinical psychologists as direct-access providers. Medicare and Medicaid, though, have been major obstacles. However, in the Omnibus Budget Reconciliation Act of 1989, major recognition of psychological services was achieved, to allow psychologists to be reimbursed independently in all Medicare settings.

Despite what seemed a clear-cut victory, the Health Care Financing Administration (HCFA) began interpreting the Medicare Conditions of

Participation for hospitals as requiring overall physician responsibility for treatment. This interpretation directly contravened law in the 11 jurisdictions (10 states and the District of Columbia) that explicitly recognized psychologists' independent-provider status in hospitals, as well as in the 18 states where the law is silent, but did not prohibit psychological practice in hospitals. However, on October 31, 1994, the Social Security Amendments of 1994, by amending Section 1861 (e)(4), struck "physician" and inserted "physician, except that a patient receiving qualified psychologist services . . . may be under the care of a clinical psychologist with respect to such services to the extent permitted under State law."

This recent legislation resolved a problem for any hospital with psychologists on its staff that was federally certified, a requirement to gain federal reimbursement for services to Medicare or Medicaid patients. Because it was not practical for hospitals to only admit non-Medicare/Medicaid patients, the prior HCFA Conditions of Participation were in effect overriding state law and the problem could only be resolved at the federal level.

Part III

Quality Improvement for Psychologists Working in Hospitals and Other Health Care Facilities

7

The Evolution of Health Care
Quality Monitoring

Psychologists who work in hospitals and other health care settings recognize their responsibility to provide the best care possible. Psychologists who are based in these facilities increasingly are becoming full and active participants in the process of identifying mechanisms both to monitor and to improve the quality of care that they are offering. In this and the following chapters, we offer information intended to assist psychologists with the development of quality monitoring programs for psychological practice in hospitals and other residential treatment facilities.

A variety of marketplace and regulatory forces are driving hospitals nationwide, with their affiliated health professionals, to monitor the quality of their health care services through programs commonly known as quality assurance, continuous quality improvement (CQI), and total quality management (TQM). In 1993, at least 60% of American hospitals reportedly embraced CQI (Lewis, 1993).[4] Unprecedented and increasing demands by third-party payers, including the federal government, for the simultaneous achievement of cost containment and high-quality care have compelled the widespread establishment of these programs in hospitals and other health care facilities. The measurement of health care quality is already a prerequisite for accreditation of health care organizations by the JCAHO and is being promoted as a key component of national and state health care reform efforts.

As noted above, psychologists practicing in hospitals and other residential treatment settings increasingly are being asked to participate in efforts to monitor and improve the quality of the psychological care being provided. The chapters in this section are intended to familiarize psychologists with the terminology, general concepts, and various methodologies commonly used or developing in the field. The descriptions provided here are not meant to be comprehensive or detailed, nor are they intended as an endorsement of any one particular methodology. Psychologists, like

---

[4]It is assumed that any CQI plan for psychological services in these facilities will be adapted to conform with each facility's own comprehensive plan for monitoring and evaluating the quality of its health care services. Note that this section is not and should not be used as an exhaustive review of this subject.

other health care providers, will differ in their individual approaches. Note that advances in this field were first developed in the corporate manufacturing sector of Japan but in the United States have been adapted to many fields, including health care services.

Quality Assurance

The measurement and evaluation of health care services have evolved in several phases. In the course of this evolution, the determination of what constitutes quality care has changed, and health care facilities have adopted a variety of approaches of measuring it. Initial efforts to ensure quality in health care tended to focus on practitioners and the ways in which they worked, using process variables. After identifying specific aspects of care to study, such as what a practitioner does in a particular setting, facilities selected indicators to measure those aspects of practice. Organizations advocating for the establishment of quality assurance programs, such as JCAHO, promoted indicators based on criteria of high-risk or high-volume activities. Using preestablished frequencies for data collection and analysis, facilities then compared the actual results against thresholds. Some of these thresholds were based on actual standards, more typically from baseline performance, and others were occasionally invented. Under this system, subthreshold performance indicated poor quality. After identifying the clinician responsible for the substandard results, supervisors were expected to take corrective action.

As quality assurance monitoring grew more widespread, many individuals and organizations recognized the limitations of a system that focused on process indicators. As a result, facilities expanded their quality assurance programs to study outcomes while reducing the number of overall indicators and raising or lowering the thresholds, but the focus remained on the performance of clinicians. Two distinctive features of traditional health care quality assurance are (a) the focus on individual clinicians, known as *outliers*, to solve problems and (b) the lack of input from patients in either defining quality or measuring outcomes.

Continuous Quality Improvement

Increasing demands for cost containment by both patients and third-party payers, including the federal government, revealed certain inadequacies inherent to quality assurance programs, such as the concentration on the activities of individual clinicians and an implied guarantee of quality. Critics of the original quality assurance methodology argued that individuals do not work in a vacuum, particularly in health care, which is frequently multidisciplinary, and that quality cannot be guaranteed but can always be improved. Accordingly, CQI developed as the next generation of quality monitoring.

CQI proponents sought to expand on quality assurance by soliciting input from consumers in defining quality, rather than solely from management or outside consultants. Note that CQI does not exclude the input of experts or professionals from the process but simply focuses on consumers as the previously neglected and relevant partners in the service delivery continuum.

In addition to the multidisciplinary nature of health care, CQI proponents recognized that clinicians function within various systems in hospitals and that the success or failure of these systems has a direct impact on patient care and treatment outcomes. Accordingly, CQI includes the study of systems as well as individuals. Other basic CQI principles are that (a) decisions regarding which staff to include on quality improvement teams must be based on the individual's knowledge of the problem or issue, not based on where people work in the organization, and (b) once a problem is identified, the determination of possible causes and remedies must be driven by data collection and evaluation.

Total Quality Management

Quality assurance and CQI may be viewed as two different approaches to controlling or improving quality in clearly focused high-priority areas. In contrast, TQM is somewhat more radical. The basic philosophy behind TQM is that every aspect of the organization is integrally related to all other aspects. The focus of TQM extends beyond monitoring individual projects or systems and, instead, addresses the management style of the organization as a whole. TQM is thus conceptualized more as a management style or philosophy that is sponsored by the organization's leadership to promote an environment supportive of continual improvement for the benefit of the organization's "customers." The health care customer includes not only patients but also purchasers of services, fiscal intermediaries, regulatory bodies, and, at times, the providers themselves. TQM is premised on the belief that many negative (or less positive) outcomes can be more efficiently addressed by systems improvements than by the corrective actions directed at individual staff. TQM is designed to empower first-line personnel to identify and correct these systems errors.

Note that there is nothing inherent in the methodologies of CQI or TQM that prevents or discourages other useful approaches to quality improvement. Most health care facilities that use these approaches continue to utilize selected monitoring and evaluation indicators, peer review, and other approaches specific to individual disciplines or departments.

Performance Improvement

Borrowing from all three of the above mentioned methodologies, JCAHO (1996), in its *Comprehensive Accreditation Manual for Hospitals*, recommends performance improvement as the basis of a comprehensive approach to quality care. (Other elements are process design, performance measurement, and performance assessment.) JCAHO suggests that organizations approach quality from the unique perspective of the mission and vision of the organization. Performance improvement begins with assessment of design, function, and expectations. This assessment in turn guides process design and measurement. Assessment, design, and measurement all contribute to the development of performance-improvement activities and their ongoing evaluation.

8

General Guidelines

The purpose of this chapter is to suggest a framework for developing a quality improvement program specific to psychological services in hospitals and other residential treatment settings. This chapter provides a series of general guidelines designed to maximize the potential of such a program and promote efficiency. Five preliminary general guidelines have been adapted primarily from the work of Jospe, Schueman, and Troy (1991). In addition, selected guidelines developed by JCAHO are presented because, as the primary overseer of quality in health care organizations across the country, JCAHO plays a major role in shaping facilities' quality review and improvement programs.

Criteria

Defining Quality

There is no single definition of quality. In a traditional quality assurance program, providers determine what constitutes quality care. However, a key feature of TQM is that the customer contributes to the definition of quality and that quality is not defined by the provider's credentials alone. Under this approach, each institution will have different customers, and therefore, the definition of the quality of patient care will vary considerably. Including the customer in the process of defining quality may help to alleviate the problem of selecting among competing definitions offered by various practitioners or professional disciplines.

Multiple Measures

The assessment of quality is best achieved by using multiple measures. Focusing on multiple aspects of the health care delivery system is the process most likely to reveal both its strengths and weaknesses.

Improvement

Quality should be monitored to improve services, not just to penalize an errant provider. To be successful, a program requires the cooperation of its health care providers. The poor reception accorded the first and second generation quality assurance programs indicates that a process that seeks primarily to punish substandard care of individuals is less likely to elicit the support of health care providers than a process that strives for ways to improve performance. To this end, the program should seek to identify systems errors as well as problematic individual activities. Subsequent corrective actions should be geared toward improving performance.

Administration

The administrative burden should be kept to a minimum. To reduce the amount of paperwork and duplication, a quality improvement program focused on psychological services should be fully integrated with the existing hospital-wide system. To maximize the potential of such a program, indicators should monitor both regularly occurring activities and high-risk events, and results should be shared with the hospital-wide program. Programs that create substantially more paperwork, that duplicate efforts already being performed, or that fail to communicate critical information are neither efficient nor effective.

Work Product Reviewed

Only representative samples of work should be reviewed. A quality improvement program is meaningful only if it is able to evaluate how a system or a provider is actually functioning. Permitting providers, for example, to select their own work for review will create an inherently biased picture.

Selected JCAHO Guidelines

Both private organizations, such as CARF, and government agencies, such as the HCFA, now survey health care delivery systems. JCAHO, however, appears to be at the forefront in this area. Accordingly, psychologists who are devising quality improvement programs for their particular facilities would be well advised to master the JCAHO requirements.

JCAHO describes its overall mission as the improvement of quality in health care provided to the public. To ensure uniformity in the quality of health care services provided by hospitals, JCAHO has established certain standards, which are regularly revised and published on an annual basis. Compliance with these standards is necessary for accreditation by

JCAHO, which is often a prerequisite for hospital licensure and reimbursement by both private and public third-party payers. These standards directly affect the practice of psychology and other professions in hospitals, detailing (a) what types of documentation staff are required to provide, (b) the manner in which information is recorded and communicated, and (c) how patients, generally, must be treated during their stay in the hospital.

As part of the mission to improve quality, JCAHO has established specific standards for quality improvement activities. In its *Comprehensive Accreditation Manual for Hospitals*, for example, JCAHO mandates that each hospital maintain a process for performance improvement. The JCAHO standards are now organized along the following functional dimensions: (a) the patient-focused functions, such as assessment and care of patients; (b) organizational functions, such as leadership and management of information; and (c) structures with functions, such as governance and medical staff. JCAHO now requires a performance-improvement project in each functional area.

Under these standards, each facility or organization must have a quality improvement plan consistent with its mission and vision for the future. This plan must be based on the needs of patients as well as staff. JCAHO expects that facilities also will rely on other sources of information with which to compare their results, such as existing research, practice guidelines, and reference databases. JCAHO considers the measurement of performance to be central to all quality improvement activities, for both processes and outcomes. JCAHO continues to require data collection activities in specific areas, such as autopsy results.

It is readily apparent that the standards require facilities to collect a great deal of data, to evaluate the data, and to follow through with specific performance-improvement activities. Nevertheless, the standards permit a wide degree of latitude as to the manner in which facilities and practitioners will do so.

9

Primary Components of Quality in the Delivery of Psychological Services in Hospitals and Other Health Care Settings

Quality improvement programs in health care services tend to address specific aspects of care. A number of components related to mental health care in particular have been identified by JCAHO and have been incorporated into the performance-improvement standards of the JCAHO *Comprehensive Accreditation Manual for Hospitals*. The components provide goals for the development of programs as well as a framework for the selection of criteria and indicators. Indicators are usually chosen because they monitor high-risk or high-volume activities.

This chapter summarizes six major components of care that are often used in the development of hospital-based quality improvement programs and provides examples of how they are applied in the quality-monitoring process. Please note that the descriptions listed below do not represent an endorsement by APA of any one particular component of care.

Accessibility of Care

Accessibility is defined as the ease with which patients can obtain the care they need when they need it. A number of indicators address access to care from a variety of perspectives. Examples of accessibility include, but are not limited to, whether patients are being referred appropriately, admitted appropriately, and assessed by a clinician with the appropriate level of training, all within a reasonable time period.

Accessibility is also defined by the Americans With Disabilities Act of 1990 (ADA) as the ability of individuals with disabilities to receive care in accordance with their special needs. The requirements of the ADA should be reviewed and incorporated into any program.

Appropriateness of Care

Appropriateness of care addresses whether the correct care is being provided. A number of indicators are available to assess the appropriateness of care, such as whether the treatment is consistent with the diagnosis reached during the psychological assessment. Similarly, the amount of treatment being provided or the degree of restriction ordered in comparison with the diagnosis and documentation on the patient's chart is another measurement tool.

Continuity of Care

In monitoring the delivery of psychological services, continuity of care is a critical component. Continuity of care refers to the delivery of care and the degree to which various aspects of care are being coordinated among psychologists and other practitioners across transitions in treatment (e.g., outpatient to inpatient to aftercare), departments, organizations, and time. Assessments of continuity are appropriate from the referral stage through discharge. Whether treatment orders are being followed is one example of continuity.

Effectiveness and Efficacy of Care

Care may be evaluated for both effectiveness and efficacy. Effectiveness is the degree to which care is provided correctly and affects the outcome. Efficacy is the degree to which a service's potential is maximized. Whether a particular service is performed without error is one example of effectiveness of care. Whether a patient has been referred for treatment to the least restrictive setting from which he or she can benefit the most is an example of the efficacy of care.

Patient Safety

The safety of the care environment is the degree to which the hospital environment is free from hazards to the patients residing there. A number of indicators monitor whether patients are being cared for safely. For example, whether they are injured by an unsafe aspect of the hospital's physical plant is one measure of patient safety.

Viewpoint of the Customer

In the current health care climate, the viewpoint of the customer is widely perceived as a critical measure of quality, one that is increasingly being relied on by hospitals. It is the degree to which patients, purchasers of services, fiscal intermediaries, and regulatory bodies are satisfied with the care provided. In the case of patients, for example, a program may wish to monitor the degree to which patients are included in the decision-making process. One example of customer satisfaction may be the number of complaints registered by patients. Note, however, that in the mental health field a patient's level of satisfaction may be affected by the actual treatment process and may not always be the most accurate measure. Other indicators will need to be examined as well.

10 _____

Fundamental Elements of a Quality Improvement Program for Psychologists in Hospitals and Other Health Care Settings

This chapter describes the fundamental elements of a successful quality improvement program and proposes possible indicators. Indicators can be selected for their application to various psychological services, but they also can be chosen for their relevance to any one of the six components or goals identified in the previous section. This chapter addresses measures that can be taken preemptively to assist in the provision of high-quality psychological services as well as indicators that can be used to monitor actual performance. All of the items were selected for their ability to fulfill at least one of the six identified goals across different psychological services. Samples of indicators for specific psychological services are provided in Appendix B.

Credentialing, Privileging, and Peer Review

Every program should include a process to ensure that members of the psychology staff are competent to provide care (credentialing) and do not provide services outside their competency (privileging). By establishing these processes, a hospital may be able to prevent unnecessary and easily avoidable occurrences of substandard treatment and other services. It is also essential that the program include a mechanism for peer review of problematic activities as they arise. All of these systems are designed to achieve maximum patient safety, appropriateness of care, effectiveness of care, and customer satisfaction. Finally, credentialing, privileging, and peer review procedures need to be established in accordance with hospital bylaws, state law, and JCAHO standards.

Credentialing

Credentialing typically involves evaluating a practitioner's basic qualifications for practice on the basis of prior education, training and experience, and documentation of credentials.

Privileging

Privileging, on the other hand, is a process for evaluating not only a practitioner's qualifications for the practice of specific techniques on the basis of prior education, training, experience, and state law but also the practitioner's level of competence. The privileging process typically includes the delineation of specific procedures to grant clinical privileges and the establishment of training and experience criteria for the granting of additional privileges to perform specific procedures. Practitioners who are granted clinical privileges are able to practice those modalities independently; other nonprivileged providers may be allowed to perform those same modalities under supervision, depending on the hospital's governing rules and bylaws.

Peer Review

Peer review is a service provided by professional associates to assess the appropriateness of the treatment goals and processes and to establish for the payer that treatment is medically or psychologically necessary and appropriate. It is also a process designed to enhance practitioner competence by the routine monitoring and evaluation of practitioners' activities.

Peer review committees for psychologists may take on two different forms. Psychologists operating within the hospital structure may elect to establish a committee solely composed of psychologists or a multidisciplinary committee, depending in part on the hospital's bylaws. In either case, the committee would in all likelihood report to a facility-wide quality-improvement department. A separate and distinct committee consisting of only psychologists has the advantage of ensuring self-evaluation for the profession. Psychologists who serve on a multidisciplinary peer review committee, however, may experience greater difficulty in developing a group of indicators specific to psychology and maintaining psychologists' independence within their scope of practice. In this instance, a first-level peer review process consisting of only psychologists should be considered.

Once a committee structure has been established, a chairperson and committee members must be appointed. The committee chair should retain overall authority and responsibility for all quality-monitoring and improvement matters involving psychologists at the hospital. In turn, the committee membership should reflect the diversity of psychological programs and services offered at the hospital. Providing representation for all psychological programs and services will ensure that appropriate psychological tasks within the hospital are adequately sampled and monitored and will allow assessment of common functions across all programs as well as unique functions within a specific program.

Occurrence Screening

Occurrence screening is the process of monitoring treatment at selected points. High-volume indicators often are particularly good indicators of quality because they are easily assessed and monitored. High-risk factors are also important to study because they ensure that known problematic areas are being regularly evaluated. For example, in all medical settings the use of medication, regardless of the medical specialty or program, is routinely found to be a high-risk area. It is important that similar problem areas in the delivery of psychological services are identified as well.

The indicators listed below are examples of indicators commonly used to monitor the quality of health care services, in particular mental health care. They are designed to focus on the clinical outcomes, because the ultimate goal of quality improvement is to evaluate psychology's contribution to patient care. Throughout this section, it should be recognized that not all occurrences are within the exclusive control of the psychologist. Unusual or problematic occurrence levels may or may not be indicative of the treating psychologist's performance.

1. Patient complaints. Monitoring patient complaints relates to the goal of customer satisfaction.
2. Scheduling problems. Monitoring canceled or late appointments addresses the combined goals of accessibility and customer satisfaction.
3. Discrimination. Monitoring provider selection of patients for discrimination on the basis of age, gender, race, ethnicity, national origin, religion, sexual orientation, disability, language, and socioeconomic status addresses the goal of accessibility. Section 1.10 of the APA (1992) "Ethical Principles" prohibits psychologists from engaging in unfair discrimination on the basis of these factors or any other factor proscribed by law. However, psychologists also are required by Section 1.04 of the APA "Ethical Principles" to practice only within the boundaries of their competence. In treating patients with unique characteristics, such as persons with disabilities, these two ethical mandates may conflict.

Providers also should take note of the Americans With Disabilities Act of 1990 (ADA). The ADA generally requires that health care practitioners, such as psychologists, provide reasonable accommodation of patients' disabilities and equivalent services. Psychologists who are asked to treat patients with disabilities should seek legal guidance if they have questions or concerns, because the law in this area is quite complex. Recent case law, for example, suggests that in the mental health field in particular, where the provider does not have experience in treating patients with a particular disability, the provider may not have to provide treatment.

Diagnostic Errors

Monitoring diagnoses for unrepresentative occurrences of diagnostic categories or treatment techniques (e.g., each patient diagnosed with the same problem or provided the same treatment) relates to appropriateness of care and will also affect efficacy of care. It should be recognized, however, that some psychologists specialize in a particular treatment area, and therefore, this indicator may not reveal diagnostic errors.

Record Keeping

Examining provider records for proper documentation addresses goals such as appropriateness, continuity, efficacy, and safety of patient care.

Patient Confidentiality

Monitoring providers and hospitals for violations of patient confidentiality addresses the goals of customer satisfaction and patient safety, in addition to state laws and health care providers' ethical obligations.

Privileging

Monitoring providers and hospitals for violations of privilege status (e.g., providing treatment without supervision in an area for which the psychologist is not privileged) promotes goals such as appropriateness, effectiveness, efficacy, and patient safety.

Prescribed Treatments

Monitoring providers for use of more restrictive environments and treatments without documentation that less severe methods have been tried and were ineffective addresses the goals of appropriateness and efficacy of patient care.

Informed Consent and Right to Refuse

Monitoring instances of inadequate informed consent and failure to respect a patient's refusal of treatment, at a minimum, addresses the goal of customer satisfaction.

Time-Based Performance Measures

Using indicators of timeliness is another way to evaluate performance. In some instances, the provision of high-quality psychological care depends on functions or tasks being performed within a specified or limited time frame. Timely performance of these tasks helps promote the goal of accessibility of care. A number of tasks for which time periods may be established and monitored are listed below:

1. Admission and patient evaluation. A time limit may be established for conducting patient evaluations on admission.
2. Documentation of treatment plan. A time limit may be established for documenting an intended course of treatment in a patient's medical chart.
3. Communication. A time limit may be established for disseminating information to all members of the multidisciplinary treatment team, the patient and family members, and other relevant parties.

Frequency-Based Performance Measures

Monitoring the frequency of occurrences is also a useful measurement tool that cuts across functions and services. The frequency indicators provided below may reveal systems errors or individual performance problems. Again, it should be recognized that unusual frequencies are not always in the exclusive control of the treating psychologist.

1. Readmissions. Number of patients readmitted (within a designated period of time) from discharge.
2. Patient requests. Number of patients requesting a different psychologist.
3. Amount of treatment. Number of patients by diagnostic category who have been seen for more than the recommended number of sessions.
4. Medication. Number of patients placed on specific medication without adequate documentation of meeting criteria for that drug (e.g., neurovegetative signs for use of antidepressant).
5. Goals. Number of patients who do not attain expected goals.
6. Suicides. Number of suicides or suicide attempts.
7. Assaults. Number of instances of self-mutilation and assault.
8. Drug and alcohol usage. Number of patients who continue usage of addictive substances after discharge.
9. Patient and staff injuries. Number of injuries to both patients and staff.

Evaluating Psychological Services Within the Hospital System

Once preventative measures have been taken and indicators have been established, the data must be collected and analyzed. To facilitate appropriate review of the data, thresholds (e.g., 100%, 95%, or 90% compliance) must be set. For example, a standard can be established that 75% of all initial consults must be completed within 48 hours of admission. If more than 25% of initial consults are conducted after 48 hours of admission, this information would indicate the need for further review.

Review of the data collected in a quality-improvement program for a hospital or other residential treatment facility typically is a task assigned to the department chair or the chair's designee, who should be a psychologist skilled in the interpretation of such data. The reviewer then reports the findings to the hospital quality-improvement department, Medical Executive Committee, or both.

Coordination of the interpretation of such data with the facility's general quality-improvement program is critical because it is clear that some of the indicators listed earlier go beyond the scope of psychologists' sole control. In many cases, the reviewer will be required to assess the interactions between psychology and other mental health disciplines. It is also possible that some indicators, such as timeliness of certain tasks around admission, treatment, and discharge, as well as the evaluation and management of the suicidal or homicidal patient, are generic indicators that will also be monitored for physicians and nurses. It may well be that the generic screen indicators collected centrally may prove informative.

It is also clear that the indicators described earlier are not alone sufficient because they do not adequately address the qualitative aspects of psychological care. Qualitative review must be conducted as well.

Communicating the Findings

The results of the analysis may then be incorporated into the professional supervision process, as well as into the formal privileging process. Most important, the results must be communicated to both practitioners and to the facility's quality-improvement department. If the data indicate that the problem rests with the individual practitioner, then a plan of correction for the practitioner may need to be developed. When the plan of correction calls for a "systems fix" (e.g., inadequate staffing, inadequate monies for materials, and poorly trained paraprofessional staff to implement behavioral treatment plans) involving multiple clinical departments and higher levels of administration, this needs to be communicated to the hospital quality-improvement department. Proper communication will assist in the achievement of quality care. In this manner, a quality-improvement program can extend beyond the individual practitioner and address systemwide issues.

In developing quality-improvement programs for their facilities, psychologists may wish to consult with other facilities in their areas, rather than duplicating efforts already under way elsewhere. Multiple programs and levels of expertise exist within each community in which psychologists practice. Many facilities, through a "cross-fertilization process" of sharing experiences, routinely provide plans that have been adapted from or are hybrids of materials from other facilities. In some states, a clearinghouse or additional resources within state associations, that will make this process much easier, may exist.

It is hoped that this section will provide the necessary guidance to help facilitate the development and implementation of a solid and effective quality-improvement program unique to the delivery of psychological services within the hospital setting. It is also hoped that this process will lead to enhanced and improved patient care.

References

American Psychiatric Association. (1994). *Diagnostic and statistical manual of mental disorders* (4th ed.). Washington, DC: Author

American Psychological Association. (1992). Ethical principles of psychologists and code of conduct. *American Psychologist, 47,* 1597–1611.

American Psychological Association, Board of Professional Affairs, Committee on Professional Standards. (1987). General guidelines for providers of psychological services. *American Psychologist, 42,* 712–723.

American Psychological Association, Board of Professional Affairs, Committee on Professional Practice. (1985). *A hospital practice primer for psychologists.* Washington, DC: American Psychological Association.

American Psychological Association, Board of Professional Affairs, Committee on Professional Practice. (1988). *Hospital practice: Advocacy issues.* Washington, DC: American Psychological Association.

Americans With Disabilities Act of 1990, 42 U.S.C.A. § 12101 *et seq.* (West 1993).

Bersoff, D. N. (1983). Hospital privileges and the antitrust laws. *American Psychologist, 38,* 1238–1242.

Copeland, B. A. (1980). Hospital privileges and staff membership for psychologists. *Professional Psychology, 11,* 676–683.

Dörken, H. (1981). Coming of age legislatively: In 21 steps. *American Psychologist, 36,* 165–173.

Dörken, H. (1983). Advocacy and the legislative process: Representation in a changing world. *American Psychologist, 38,* 1210–1215.

Dörken, H., & Carpenter, L. (1986). How state legislation opens markets for practice. In H. Dörken & Associates (Eds.), *Professional psychology in transition: Meeting today's challenge* (pp. 247–282). San Francisco: Jossey-Bass.

Dörken, H., Stapp, J., & VandenBos, G. (1986). Licensed psychologists: A decade of major growth. In H. Dörken & Associates (Eds.), *Professional psychology in transition: Meeting today's challenge* (pp. 3–19). San Francisco: Jossey-Bass.

Dörken, H., VandenBos, G., Henke, C., Cummings, N. A., & Pallak, M. (1993). Impact of law and regulation on professional practice and use of mental health services: An empirical analysis. *Professional Psychology: Research and Practice, 24,* 256–265.

Employee Retirement Income Security Act of 1974, 29 U.S.C. § 1001 *et seq.*

Federal Employees' Compensation Act of 1916, 39 U.S.C. § 742 (1916) as amended.

Health Maintenance Organization Development Act of 1973, 42 U.S.C. § 300e *et seq.*

Joint Commission on Accreditation of Healthcare Organizations. (1996). *Comprehensive accreditation manual for hospitals.* Chicago: Author.

Jospe, M., Schueman, S. & Troy, W. (1991). Quality assurance and the clinical health psychologist: A programmatic approach. In J. J. Sweet, R. H. Rozensky, & S. M. Tovian (Eds.), *Handbook of clinical psychology in medical settings* (pp. 95–112). New York: Plenum.

Kurz, R. B., Fuchs, M., Dabek, R. F., Kurtz, S. M. S., & Helfrich, W. T. (1982). Characteristics of predoctoral internships in professional psychology. *American Psychologist, 37,* 1213–1220.

Lewis, A. (1993). Too many managers: Major threat to CQI in hospitals. *Quality Review Bulletin, 19,* 95–101.

Omnibus Budget Reconciliation Act of 1989, Pub. L. No. 101-239, § 103 Stat. (1989).

Pallak, M. S., Cummings, N., Dörken, H., & Henke, C. (1994). Medical costs, Medicaid, and managed mental health treatment: The Hawaii study. *Managed Care Quarterly, 2,* 64–70.

Pion, G., Kohout, J., & VandenBos, G. R. (1990). Human resources in mental health. In R. Manderscheid & M. Sonnenschein (Eds.), *Mental health United States 1990* (DHHS Publication No. ADM 90-1708). Washington, DC: U.S. Government Printing Office.

Reaves, R. P. (1984). *The law of professional licensing and certification*. Charlotte, NC: Publications for Professionals.

Rozensky, R. H. (1997). Medical or professional staff membership and participation in rural hospitals. In J. A. Morris (Ed.), *Practicing psychology in rural settings: Hospital privileges and collaborative care* (pp. 19–36). Washington, DC: American Psychological Association.

Schlesinger, H., Mumford, E., Patrick IV, C., & Sharfstein, S. (1983). Mental health treatment and medical care utilization in a fee-for-service system: Outpatient treatment following the onset of a chronic disease. *American Journal of Public Health, 73,* 422–429.

Sciara, A. (1983). *Hospital privileges training course*. Unpublished manuscript.

Social Security Act of 1994, Pub. L. No. 103-432, § 108 Stat. (1994).

Tanney, F. (1985). Hospital privileges legislation and the political process. *Psychotherapy in Private Practice, 3,* 107–114.

Annotated Bibliography

Albright, D. (1986). School liaison: Evaluation and treatment. *Psychiatric Hospital, 17*, 133–136.

> The author argues for the development of a psychiatric assessment service for school-age children within hospitals as a cost-effective source of revenue and a referral base. It is suggested that outpatient services should include evaluations, treatment, and consultation with school officials regarding treatment. Consultative services may consist of education of school staff about psychological disorders and assistance in the development of school assistance programs.

Arnett, J., Martin, R., Streiner, D., & Goodman, J. (1987). Hospital psychology in Canada. *Canadian Psychology, 28*, 161–171.

> The authors examine Canadian hospital psychology in terms of the existing organizational models, professional practices, academic activities, and professional orientations of hospital psychologists, in a survey of 340 hospitals. Results revealed that psychologists were active clinically and academically in Canadian hospitals in a wide variety of health care areas, in addition to traditional mental health areas. In the majority of hospitals, psychologists were organized in independent departments of psychology or behavioral science, although physician influence appeared to be a strong factor in practice. Medical staff membership and academic appointments for hospital psychologists were relatively low. Recommendations for the future development of hospital psychology in Canada are outlined.

Barlow, D. (1994). Psychological interventions in the era of managed competition. *Clinical Psychology: Science and Practice, 1*, 109–122.

> Outcome studies show the effectiveness of specific psychological treatments with specific disorders and note that "the problem of gaining acceptance for psychological treatment is not one of effectiveness. The problem is public relational and . . . political." Evidence shows that psychological treatment is effective for alcohol abuse and dependence, depression, panic disorder, agoraphobia, generalized anxiety disorder, obsessive–compulsive disorder, and schizophrenia (the latter in combination with medication). Cognitive–behavioral therapy and interpersonal therapy are both effective on follow-up with bulimia. "There is no drug treatment with proven effectiveness available for this serious eating disorder." Report on dialectical behavior therapy in the long-term treatment of borderline personality disorder found that fewer individuals attempted suicide over a 1-year period and those "receiving DBT were hospitalized an average of 8.4 days a year as compared to 38.8 days . . . for control subjects."

Belar, C., Deardorff, W., & Kelly, K. (1987). *The practice of clinical health psychology*. Oxford, England: Pergamon Press.

> This book is focused on clinical health psychology practice issues related to treatment in outpatient and inpatient settings. The issues dealt with (e.g., core content, professional roles, ethics, malpractice, assessment, and intervention) represent those areas found to be of special importance in clinical practice. Throughout the book the authors have attempted to identify common pitfalls in practice and to provide ideas on how to effectively manage these areas.

Bersoff, D. (1983). Hospital privileges and antitrust laws. *American Psychologist, 38*, 1232–1237.

> The author discusses the antitrust implications of denying hospital privileges to psychologists as a class within the context of a statute that was currently before the District of Columbia Council. Section 8 of the statute would prohibit hospitals from categorically denying staff privileges to psychologists and certain other health care providers and would require hospitals to make decisions on the basis of individual qualifications. The article highlights the advantages that passage of such statute would produce and suggests the legal theories that could be used to challenge practices in other jurisdictions on antitrust grounds if these jurisdictions are not yet considering legislation similar to that in the District of Columbia.

Bleiberg, J., Ciulla, R., & Katz, B. (1991). Psychological components of rehabilitation programs for brain-injured and spinal-cord-injured patients. In J. Sweet, R. Rozensky, & S. Tovian (Eds.), *Handbook of clinical psychology in medical settings* (pp. 375–440). New York: Plenum.

> This chapter examines clinical psychology as practiced in the rehabilitation hospital. The clinical and administrative environment of the rehabilitation hospital is described, with emphasis on how it affects the role definition and mode of practice of psychologists. Two specific populations, spinal-cord-injured and brain-injured patients, are examined to identify and illustrate the issues specific to the psychological care of each group.

Brigham, D., & Toal, P. O. (1991). The use of imagery in a multimodal psychoneuroimmunology program for cancer and other chronic diseases. In Kunzendorf (Ed.), *Mental imagery* (pp. 193–198). New York: Plenum.

> The Getting Well program at Orlando General Hospital has translated the literature in the area of psychoneuroimmunology into viable life techniques for people with cancer and other chronic diseases such as multiple sclerosis, lupus, HIV, irritable bowel syndrome, rheumatoid arthritis, and neurological dysfunctions. This intensive adjunctive inpatient program draws from all areas of cognitive–behavioral medicine to immerse the participant in new ways of living and perception of the world. Imagery provides the backbone for the program and is the focus of this chapter.

Carpenter, P. (1989). Establishing the role of the pediatric psychologist in a university medical center–based oncology service. *Journal of Training and Practice in Professional Psychology, 3,* 21–28.

> Training psychologists to assume both clinical and academic roles in pediatric medical settings is viewed as a professional priority. This article describes the author's experiences in establishing the role of the pediatric psychologist in a university medical center–based oncology unit as a member of the health care team. The advantages as well as the pitfalls are discussed. A model is outlined for the training and supervision of psychologists to assume positions in pediatric subspecialties.

Charlop, M., Parrish, J., Fenton, L., & Cataldo, M. (1987). Evaluation of hospital-based outpatient pediatric psychology services. *Journal of Pediatric Psychology, 12,* 485–503.

> The authors analyze the service characteristics of 100 patients (aged 1–12 years) referred consecutively to a pediatric psychology clinic, in terms of patient and problem characteristics, recommended treatments, clinical outcome, and consumer satisfaction. Results provide an example of quantitatively documenting clinic efficacy and deficiency, an activity increasingly necessary for the survival of pediatric psychology services in a financially burdened health care system.

Clayson, D., & Mensh, I. (1987). Psychologists in medical schools: The trials of emerging political activism. *American Psychologist, 42,* 859–862.

> Psychology in medical education has a history of about 75 years. Although there has been communication among psychologists in this applied field, such communication has been informal, except for a series of conferences during the past 40 years. The Association of Medical School Professors of Psychology now has formal status and is affiliated with the Association of American Medical Colleges, the organization that is primarily responsible for the direction of medical education in the United States. Growth in numbers from relatively few faculty members to approximately 3,000 is a positive direction. Yet, the independence of the field continues to be a problem, although contributions by psychologists to medical education have been clearly demonstrated. Data from a 1984 survey of 3,600 respondent hospitals show the proportions granting staff membership or privileges by profession.

Cummings, J. (1992). Psychologists in the medical–surgical setting: Some reflections. *Professional Psychology: Research and Practice, 23,* 76–79.

> This article reflects on the early entry of clinical and counseling psychology into the general medical hospital setting in the 1950s and 1960s. Drawing largely from 3.5 decades as a Department of Veterans Affairs psychologist (mainly in the areas of tuberculosis and end stage renal disease), the author describes problems and contributions associated with psychology's entry into this new arena. Not only did these

involve providing direct patient services at the bedside; just as much, they involved clarifying psychological health concepts, the training of patients and their families in taking the most active roles in their own treatment, and the professional relationships between psychologists and their new colleagues in the medical and surgical wards.

Dörken, H. (1981). The hospital practice of psychology. *Professional Psychology*, *12*, 599–605.

The California laws that support and enable clinical psychologists to practice in hospitals and provide other formal recognition of such practice are outlined, including favorable attorney general opinions. Noted are laws requiring that diagnostic and treatment services be provided only by licensed health professionals, that denial or revocation of staff privileges be reported to licensing boards, that the decisions and reasons to deny staff privileges be discoverable, and that the Nurse Practice Act be amended to include clinical psychologists among those who may issue nursing orders. Survey data at that time, when projected nationally, indicated that the number of licensed psychologists holding appointments to the organized medical staff of a hospital was approximately 6,800.

The concluding paragraph is pertinent today: "The laws . . . in California . . . have emphasized organized models of practice . . . because of a . . . realization of the near term future. We have already entered the beginning stages of the industrialization of healthcare. This evolution/revolution will see organized models of care rapidly replace the cottage industry of solo practice . . . survival will depend on our ability to create psychological health systems . . . and to be colleagues, even owners of multidisciplinary health facilities."

Dörken, H. (1988). Psychotherapy in the marketplace: CHAMPUS 1986. *Psychotherapy*, *25*, 387–392.

From 1975 to 1986 there has been an increase in the number of professionals providing mental health services, with a continuing penetration into this market by psychologists, although with wide variation among states. Individual hourly psychotherapy accounted for about 75% of all outpatient visits and about 50% of inpatient visits. Only 3% of psychiatrist visits, in- or outpatient, were for services that could be provided only by a physician, underscoring the overlap among and competition between the mental health professions.

Dörken, H. (1989). Hospital practice as gatekeeper to continuity of care: CHAMPUS mental health services, 1980–1987. *Professional Psychology: Research and Practice*, *20*, 419–420.

Although outpatient and inpatient mental health services may have been separate realms of care in the 1940s and even well into the 1960s, dual-level care is common today. Psychology and physician practice acts define the scope of practice but place no restraints on locus of care. Data from CHAMPUS clearly show that about 10% of outpatients and about 60% of inpatients, the majority, also receive overlapping care at the alternative level. Any movement to constrain practice to one location disrupts both continuity of care and the ability of a practitioner to compete in the marketplace. Not having the standing to practice in hospitals is a handicap.

Dörken, H. (1993). The hospital private practice of psychology: CHAMPUS 1981–1991. *Professional Psychology: Research and Practice, 24,* 409–417.

This article reviews and analyzes CHAMPUS inpatient data from 1981 to 1991. Utilization data are presented by state, year, and profession for inpatient visits. There has been a moderate but progressive growth in the proportion of inpatient visits provided by psychologists over these years, from 3.3% to 19.4%, nationally. In terms of beneficiaries receiving some psychological services, the proportion increased from 7.2% to 26.5%. Visit level in 1991 was highest in Texas, at 30.5%, and least in Georgia, at 12.7%, among the nine states detailed. Psychiatry has seen a 20% drop in the proportion of inpatient visits it has rendered over these years, and fewer psychiatrists provided CHAMPUS services in 1991 than in 1981. These data reflect the fact that the private practice of psychology in hospitals has gained increasing recognition.

Dörken, H. (1994). The CHAMPUS Reform Initiative in Hawaii: Reestablishing a medical monopoly. *Professional Psychology: Research and Practice, 25,* 102–105.

This study examines the effect of the CHAMPUS Reform Initiative (CRI) in Hawaii. Data are presented from 1986 to 1991 on the professions involved, outpatient and inpatient services rendered, and psychotherapy fees by profession. This "medical gatekeeper" model of managed care, based on a system of referral to specialist services by primary-care physicians and developed by a Hawaiian medical group, yielded predictable results. Whereas psychologists had been the dominant providers of outpatient mental health services since 1980 and had a minor presence in inpatient services, the implementation of CRI resulted in psychiatrists becoming the dominant outpatient provider and psychologists essentially being eliminated from hospital practice. These results should alert psychologists to the danger of extinction from medical monopolies. Managed care will add further change and future uncertainties that few practitioners will escape. The scope and import of these changes are discussed.

Dörken, H., & Webb, J. (1979). The hospital practice of psychology: An interstate comparison. *Professional Psychology, 10,* 619–630.

Clinical privileges among psychologists are more common than membership in the organized medical/professional staff of hospitals. Forty percent are on an informal basis. This article is an interstate comparison (California, Ohio, Illinois, Texas, Florida, and New York). It notes some consistent trends and explainable differences, which appear to be the consequence of restraint of trade or boycott rather than disinterest in hospital practice on the part of psychologists.

Dörken, H., Webb, J. T., & Zaro, J. (1982). Hospital practice of psychology resur-
veyed: 1980. *Professional Psychology, 13*, 814–829.

> This article summarizes psychologists' attempts to engage the JCAHO
> and reviews the service delivery patterns of psychologists and psychi-
> atrists. The nature of hospital practice by psychologists in 10 states is
> reviewed. The article is important for its delineation of privileges for
> psychologists in a hospital setting and its evaluation of the importance
> of hospital privileges and practice for psychologists in the future.

Drotar, D. (1987). Psychological consultation in medical settings: Challenges and
constraints. In J. R. McNamara & M. A. Appel (Eds.), *Critical issues, developments, and trends in professional psychology, Vol. 3. Professional psychology
update* (pp. 80–111). New York: Praeger.

> The author describes the practice of psychological consultation/liaison
> in medical settings and implications for psychology as a profession;
> notes setting differences among community hospitals, teaching hospi-
> tals, ambulatory settings, and rehabilitation centers; and outlines the
> prospects for productive collaboration with physicians and how to train
> psychological consultants for program development and survival and
> growth in medical settings.

Dunn, R. (1986). General hospital psychology. *Canadian Psychology, 27*, 44–50.

> This article reviews major developments in the practice of hospital psy-
> chology, focusing on four current influences on hospital psychologists
> —the deinstitutionalization of chronic mental patients, the emergence
> of health psychology and behavioral medicine, the changing nature
> of hospitals, and the pursuit of increased autonomy by general hospi-
> tal psychologists. A matrix within which to conceptualize and evaluate
> hospital-based psychological services is presented.

Eisenberg, M., & Jansen, M. (1987). Rehabilitation psychologists in medical settings: A unique subspecialty or a redundant one? *Professional Psychology: Research and Practice, 18*, 475–478.

> A critique of the literature addressing functions of rehabilitation psy-
> chologists in medical settings was accomplished to determine the range
> of roles typically assumed by them. Although this search yielded rela-
> tively few citations that clearly outlined duties and functions commonly
> undertaken by psychologists in medical settings, it did provide evidence
> that many use a behavioral framework and that psychologists' incor-
> poration of new technologies, such as biofeedback, has helped to main-
> stream them into medical practice. In addition, the current emphasis
> placed on cost containment suggests that many of the treatment mo-
> dalities practiced by rehabilitation psychologists will be increasingly
> used in medical settings.

Enright, M. (1985). The psychologist in medical arts practice and small hospitals.
Psychotherapy in Private Practice, 3, 9–21.

The author discusses possible roles of private-practice psychologists working in consultation with a medical arts practice or a small hospital. Issues addressed include (a) identification of medical patients in need of psychological services, (b) the development of professional relationships and reciprocal referral arrangements with physicians, (c) the psychologist's role in the small general hospital, (d) advantages of working in a medical arts practice, and (e) psychological intervention with physicians. It is concluded that there is a place for psychological consultation in the practice of all medical subspecialties and in many different milieus. The author's personal experience suggests that a meaningful and rewarding professional relationship awaits the psychologist in an equal and cooperative role with other medical practitioners, both in the small hospital and in a medical arts practice.

Enright, M., Resnick, R., DeLeon, P., Sciara, A. D., & Tanney, F. (1990). The practice of psychology in hospital settings. *American Psychologist, 45,* 1059–1065.

> Psychologists are taking the lead to ensure that consumers have full access to behavioral science knowledge in America's hospitals. This article recaps the development of psychology's position in hospitals and explores the variety of current and prospective roles of psychologists in inpatient health care.

Enright, M., Resnick, R., Ludwigsen, K., & DeLeon, P. (1993). Hospital practice: Psychology's call to action. *Professional Psychology: Research and Practice, 24,* 135–141.

> The general public has recently made demands for continuity of care in psychological services from outpatient settings to inpatient facilities and back. These demands plus three economic and structural modifications within our nation's health care arena, including the incursion of for-profit health care corporations into the health delivery industry, the 1985 JCAH decision to include nonphysician providers on hospital medical staffs, and the 1990 California Supreme Court decision (*CAPP v. Rank*) ensuring full medical staff participation by California psychologists, have opened the doors to the independent practice of psychology in hospitals, rehabilitation centers, nursing homes, and day treatment facilities. This article presents current professional realities for psychologists in hospitals and health care settings and reviews the work of the American Psychological Association in support of hospital independent practice.

Enright, M., Welch, B., Newman, R., & Perry, B. (1990). The hospital: Psychology's challenge in the 1990s. *American Psychologist, 45,* 1057–1058.

> The authors discuss the growing pressure on psychologists to take the role of attending clinician in hospital settings and describe the efforts of external forces to challenge psychology's movement into the inpatient venue. This challenge is illustrated in the recent court action of *CAPP v. Rank* (1990), which began as a challenge by psychology to the California Department of Health Services hospital regulations and developed into an attack on psychology's scope of licensure.

Fisher, W., Dorwart, R., Schlesinger, M., & Davidson, H. (1991). Contracting between public agencies and private psychiatric inpatient facilities. *Medical Care, 29,* 766–774.

> Purchasing services through contracts with private providers has become an increasingly common practice over the past 20 years. Using data from a national survey of psychiatric inpatient facilities, this article examines the extent to which psychiatric units in privately controlled general hospitals and private psychiatric specialty hospitals (*N* = 611) participate in contractual arrangements to provide services to government bodies. The findings indicate that nonprofit psychiatric specialty hospitals were more likely than other types of hospitals to enter into such contracts and that forces such as local competition and need for services were not predictors of such involvement. Contracting was shown to have a significant impact on the level of referrals a hospital accepted. These data suggest that public agencies contracting for services with private hospitals may represent a means by which "public-sector" patients may gain access to private providers. Further, this mechanism may impose sufficient structure and regulation on the acceptance of such patients, that many concerns of hospital administrators regarding patients who are costly and difficult to treat and discharge can be allayed.

Follette, W., & Cummings, N. (1967). Psychiatric services and medical utilization in a prepaid health plan setting. *Medical Care, 5,* 25–35.

> The classic and watershed study that showed that the *one interview* and *brief psychotherapy* groups (average 6.2 visits) had a subsequent significant decline in overall health care utilization, including hospital days. For the *long-term therapy* group (average 33.9 visits) psychotherapy visits supplanted medical visits, but there was a significant decline in hospital days to the health plan average. The reductions in utilization after the second-year follow-up were stable over 5 years. It was also evident that mental health users are high users of health care.

Garrick, T., & Loewenstein, R. (1989). Behavioral medicine in the general hospital. *Psychosomatics, 30,* 123–134.

> This article summarizes the impact of clinical behavioral medicine in the assessment and treatment of medical, psychophysiological, and psychosomatic problems. Specific techniques of behavioral assessment and behavioral treatment strategies, as well as some general and conceptual issues, are discussed. The illnesses for which these interventions have been useful include chronic pain, behavior disorders, asthma, and irritable bowel syndrome. Five case histories are presented.

Goldwurm, G., Rovetto, F., & Sardo, A. (1986). Towards the establishment of a behavioural medicine centre in a general hospital. *Activitas Nervosa Superior, 28,* 77–78.

> The authors discuss the creation of a behavioral medicine center in Niguarda General Hospital in Milan, Italy. Those treated are not la-

beled as psychiatric patients and do not believe that they have psychiatric disorders. Despite initial difficulties in establishing the center, it is maintained that the great potential benefit of a behavioral approach to the prevention, treatment, and rehabilitation of various psychophysical disorders is becoming increasingly evident.

Goodman, J., Goodman, M., McGrath, J., & Goldsmith, L. (1987). Quality assurance in psychological services. *Canadian Psychology, 28*, 172–179.

> The Canadian Council on Hospital Accreditation (1985) has insisted that a hospital-wide quality assurance program is essential for accreditation, and hospital departments are in various stages of quality assurance program development. The present authors review the rationale and issues (e.g., professional autonomy, malpractice, health care costs, and consumerism) that forced the development of quality assurance and some generally accepted definitions of key concepts. The current status of the Children's Hospital of Eastern Ontario Psychology Department's program of quality assurance is described, with specific reference to structure, process, and outcome criteria. Implications of quality assurance programs for the professional practice of psychology and functioning within the public hospital setting are discussed.

Gutmann, M., Sanson-Fisher, R., Christiansen, B., & Blackwell, B. (1987). Behavioral medicine programs in teaching hospitals. *Psychotherapy and Psychosomatics, 48*, 116–122.

> The authors suggest that behavioral medicine (BM) is an interdisciplinary field that combines biomedical and behavioral science knowledge and applies it to prevention, diagnosis, treatment, and rehabilitation. BM programs provide a valuable service to patients with chronic illness, psychosomatic or functional disorders, treatment noncompliance, and behavioral risk factors. BM faculty are also active in teaching and research on patient behavior, interviewing skills, health promotion and counseling, and management of chronic illnesses. It is noted that the survival of BM programs in teaching hospitals depends on their economic viability and academic status. The organization and integration of a BM program are described.

Hickling, E., Sison, G., & Holtz, J. (1985). Role of psychologists in multidisciplinary pain clinics: A national survey. *Professional Psychology: Research and Practice, 16*, 868–880.

> The authors investigate the roles and responsibilities of psychologists functioning in multidisciplinary pain clinics by surveying 116 comprehensive pain centers throughout the United States. Seventy-six surveys (65.5%) that contained analyzable data were returned. Results indicate the following: (a) Psychologists divide their time approximately equally among therapy, evaluation, and other roles; (b) the majority of all pain clinic patients are seen by the psychologist on the team; and (c) behaviorally oriented models of intervention are used most often by the psychologist. Nearly all of the psychologists used clinical interviews in

evaluation, along with the Minnesota Multiphasic Personality Inventory. Pain questionnaires, especially the Beck Depression Inventory, were also frequently used evaluative devices. Results suggest that needed skills include psychotherapy, assessment, and application of learning theory to the understanding of pain.

Holmes, J., Taylor, C., & Begun, P. (1995, March). Healthcare: PPMs are attractive alternative. *Kemper Securities Equity Roundup*, pp. 36–37.

This article reviews physician practice management (PPM) organizations as a newly emerging and growing area of health care services. The American Medical Association (AMA) reports that from 1965 to 1991 the number of physicians practicing in groups increased 550%, from 28,381 to 184,358. Also, the percentage of group physicians among total nonfederal physicians increased from 10.6% in 1961 to 32% in 1991. PPMs achieve a critical mass of physicians, so that they can diversify the financial risk in a capitated environment.

In 1993 there were 3,587 multispecialty groups, according to the AMA. PPMs, by buying out group practices under long-term agreements, can contribute economies of scale and can increase "same store sales" (clinics) by adding practitioners and ancillary service and by acquiring additional clinics/groups. This allows more flexibility in future contracting than in selling to a hospital or insurer.

Hopkin, J. (1985). Psychiatry and medicine in the emergency room. *New Directions for Mental Health Services, 28,* 47–53.

The author discusses problems related to the differentiation of medical and psychological treatment of patients seen in emergency psychiatry, considering the increasing recognition that organic and functional mental disorders show a high degree of overlap. Case vignettes of a 31-year-old man with acquired immune deficiency syndrome (AIDS) and of a 56-year-old woman showing signs of mental deterioration illustrate the importance of knowledge of the variety of conditions that could have resulted in the behavioral symptoms, the capacity to perform a diagnostic work-up under difficult conditions, and the provision of psychological support. Problems in the operation of a psychiatric emergency service that relate to an emphasis on psychosocial stress to the exclusion of medically oriented treatment are described. The need for a broad spectrum of skills in the emergency psychiatric setting is emphasized.

Janocko, K. M., & Lee, S. (1988). Ethical implications of deinstitutionalization and moves of the institutionalized elderly. *Professional Psychology: Research and Practice, 19,* 522–526.

This article focuses on the ethical issues faced by psychologists working as members of an interdisciplinary team in a psychiatric hospital in the light of the current trend and policy to deinstitutionalize. The major ethical dilemma results from psychologists' awareness of the effects of long-term institutionalization and moves on older people, as well as some of the documented adverse consequences of deinstitutionalization.

The authors review the current policy on deinstitutionalization and the literature on the effects of deinstitutionalization and relocation on older people. They also address the role of the psychologist in a hospital setting wherein there may be goals and values that conflict with those of the therapists. Possible ways to resolve this conflict of interest are explored.

Jostad, J. (1987). Some experience in psychotherapy with suicidal patients. *Acta Psychiatrica Scandinavica, 76,* 76–81.

This article outlines three prerequisites for psychodynamic psychotherapy of suicidal patients: a psychodynamic understanding, a psychotherapeutic attitude, and a psychotherapeutic method. Changes in actual relationships and self-esteem are believed to be of particular importance. The therapist must be more direct, personal, and interrogating than is the case with other types of patients, especially with regard to the suicidal fantasies and acts. The author emphasizes the importance of identifying hateful countertransference reactions in the therapist. An important aspect in consultations with hospitalized patients is to ask questions and to use direct communication about suicidal intentions and risks at ward meetings or in group work. It is also essential to address countertransference reactions in the staff. The postmortem work after a successful suicide must include fellow patients, staff members, and the family.

Kastenbaum, R. (1982). The psychologist and hospital policy. *American Psychologist, 37,* 1355–1358.

Using his own experience as a hospital director, the author discusses psychologists' unique skills that are needed in hospitals. In particular, he describes their ability to assess complex situations, to understand the constituencies and special interests involved in a hospital, to assist employees in tracking the consequences of their decisions, and to improve communication patterns.

Kiesler, C. (1991). Changes in general hospital psychiatric care, 1980–1985. *American Psychologist, 46,* 416–421.

More than 60% of all inpatient psychiatric episodes occur in general hospitals. The need for psychologists' involvement in this important area is discussed. Changes in general hospital inpatient care from 1980 to 1985 are described. These include important and controversial changes in public policy, most notably Medicare's prospective payment system. Substantial changes in the de facto system occurred in patterns of diagnosis, sites of care, and the role of third-party payers. Implications for public policy and future investigations are drawn.

Kiesler, C., & Simpkins, C. (1991). The de facto national system of psychiatric inpatient care: Piecing together the national puzzle. *American Psychologist, 46,* 579–584.

National data regarding psychiatric inpatient episodes can be viewed in two ways. The normative method surveys the "specialty mental health sector." A more inclusive method includes smaller sites (e.g., the military), all of general hospital treatment (rather than only the psychiatric unit), residential treatment centers, and other residential care. The difference between the two methods represents approximately 725,000 episodes, at a direct cost of more than $6 billion. The more inclusive analysis of the years 1980 and 1985 reveals a strong shift to the private sector and an increase in inpatient care of children and youth that might be obscured by limiting national treatment statistics to the specialty mental health sector.

Klein, N. (1990). The psychologist as admitting clinician: A single case example. *American Psychologist, 45*, 1071–1073.

An experiential view of significant issues associated with independent hospital practice for psychologists is offered through a case presentation. The example is a model of practice—in effect at a 90-bed, freestanding, inpatient facility opened in 1985—that gives psychologists full professional staff privileges.

Litwin, W., Boswell, D., & Kraft, W. (1991). Medical staff membership and clinical privileges: A survey of hospital-affiliated psychologists. *Professional Psychology: Research and Practice, 22*, 322–327.

A survey of 582 hospital-affiliated psychologists was conducted regarding the hospital clinical privileges of psychologists. Response rate was 72.2%. Results suggest that although psychologists are making progress in gaining medical staff membership and associated clinical privileges, this progress is slow. Analyses suggest that most psychologists have the privilege to conduct testing, therapy, and research independently of physicians; however, many still lack these basic privileges. In addition, other privileges such as admission, discharge, and ordering medical referrals are afforded to only a very limited number of psychologists. Psychologists are most satisfied with the full, independent level of privilege for all 18 privileges.

Ludwigsen, K. R. (Ed.). (1987). *Hospital practice in California: A manual for psychologists*. Los Angeles: Division of Clinical and Professional Psychology, California State Psychological Association.

This manual describes the grassroots efforts of California psychologists whose involvement in hospital practice has helped clarify and strengthen the role of psychology in hospital settings. Chapters address such issues as psychologists' preparation for legal rights in hospital practice, advocacy, hospitalization of patients, and the role of psychology in the general hospital. An extensive glossary appendix and list of resources make this a helpful guide for psychologists seeking hospital privileges in any state.

Ludwigsen, K. (1992). Psychologists: An essential component to hospital healthcare. *Psychotherapy in Private Practice, 10*, 145–150.

The author discusses why hospitals are making increasing use of psychological services in the 1990s. Psychologists can help hospitals through (a) reducing medical overutilization by treating patients' underlying problems, (b) treating psychological issues that are complicating factors in stress-related disorders, (c) reducing length of hospital stay, (d) reducing risk of malpractice suits, and (e) making hospital referrals. Other trends that favor increased use of psychological services by hospitals include the role of the hospital as a community resource and the shift from the disease model to the patient education model of health care.

Ludwigsen, K. (1993a). Advocacy issues in hospital practice. *Independent Practitioner, 13,* 174–176.

A pragmatic outline of useful strategy in the advocacy for hospital privileges with steps to consider hospital by hospital.

Ludwigsen, K. (1993b). Credentialing and privileging issues in hospital practice. *Register Report, 19,* 3–6.

The *National Register* has identified close to 700 hospitals at which psychologists have formal hospital staff membership (HSM) and will designate such registrants in future annual registers. (In 1994, 1,809 registrants had the HSM designation.) Underscores the importance of professional standards and current competence. Notes that there are graduated levels of responsibility reflected in levels of HSM from affiliate/allied health staff, to consulting staff, to active/courtesy staff.

Ludwigsen, K., & Albright, D. (1994). Training psychologists for hospital practice: A proposal. *Professional Psychology: Research and Practice, 25,* 241–246.

Hospital practice has become increasingly important for psychologists over the past decade. However, expanded opportunities for practice require training for competency. The authors propose developing a comprehensive, systematic, and flexible program of training for hospital practice in psychology, including graduate course work, supervised practicum experience, and opportunities for retraining. Recommendations for certification in hospital practice, credentialing and privileging, and continuing education are included.

Margolis, R., Duckro, P., & Merkel, W. (1992). Behavioral medicine: St. Louis style. *Professional Psychology: Research and Practice, 23,* 293–299.

This article describes a unique multidisciplinary division in which eight clinical programs are all administered by psychologists working in a university medical center setting. The increasingly complex environment of a university medical center is discussed in terms of academic mission, competitiveness of health care, and professional roles. The development of this division is reviewed in relation to a number of critical issues, such as organizational structure, academic versus clinical demands, business operations, and one version of a scientist/practitioner model in practice.

McGuire, T., Trupin, E., & Rothenberg, M. (1985). Survey of the utilization of psychiatrists and psychologists for hospitalized children. *Children's Health Care, 14*, 114–117.

> Ten nurses and 67 pediatricians completed a questionnaire designed to assess the disciplines involved, the availability of various personnel, teaching functions, funding of services, and perceived need for further services in providing psychosocial care to hospitalized children. Results show that psychiatrists and psychologists were used least often in all settings. Respondents from 68% of the 22 hospitals represented specifically requested more services from psychiatrists and psychologists trained in pediatric issues. Possible reasons for the underuse of psychologists and psychiatrists include (a) their high salaries may make them less cost-effective caregivers, (b) they may find it difficult to give up the financial benefits of private practice to practice in a hospital setting, (c) they may be unwilling to extend their training to include skills for consultation in pediatrics, (d) there may be resistance from medical colleagues who do not view psychology/psychiatry as "real" medicine, and (e) the area of consultation/liaison is so new that some pediatricians are not aware of what psychologists/psychiatrists have to offer.

Mickel, C. (1982). Innovative projects earning psychologists spots on hospital healthcare terms. *American Psychologist, 37*, 1350–1354.

> Innovative hospital projects initiated by psychologists include the use of video games to restore and measure mental functions in seriously injured patients, biofeedback therapy, the use of behavioral techniques to reduce and eliminate pain associated with cancer or with chemotherapy, and the monitoring of high-risk infants. While psychologists have had to fight for hospital privileges, there seems to be a slow movement toward allowing these privileges. Psychologists could also be useful in such areas as stress management, the design of special wheelchairs, and behavior modification for smokers and the obese.

Miller, W., & Hester, R. (1986). Inpatient alcoholism treatment: Who benefits? *American Psychologist, 41*, 794–805.

> Although uncontrolled studies have yielded mixed findings, 26 controlled comparisons have consistently shown no overall advantage for residential over nonresidential settings, for longer over shorter inpatient programs, or for more intensive over less intensive interventions in treating alcohol abuse. Predictor data suggest that intensive treatment may be differentially beneficial for more severely deteriorated and less socially stable individuals. The outcome of alcoholism treatment is more likely to be influenced by the content of interventions than by the settings in which they are offered. Third-party reimbursement policy should discourage the use of intensive residential models for addressing alcohol abuse when more cost-effective alternatives are available and should reinforce the use of research-supported treatment methods regardless of setting. Such policy priorities run directly counter to the current practices and financial interests of many for-profit providers.

Newman, R. (1990). Independent practice in hospitals: A cornerstone for professional legitimacy. *Hospital Progress Notes, 1*, 3–4.

> The author emphasizes that "Because the hospital setting provides a
> prototype for healthcare, independent practice in hospitals to the full
> extent of psychology licensure will ultimately determine psychology's
> stature in all settings." Cites the *CAPP v. Rank* (1990) lawsuit in Cal-
> ifornia and subsequent challenges and decisions in Washington State.
> "Once again, a question of psychology's ability to practice in hospitals
> has become a question of psychology's ability to practice independently
> in general."
>
> (The Supreme Court of California concluded June 25, 1990, "that
> under California law a hospital that admits psychologists to its staff
> may permit such psychologists to take primary responsibility for the
> admission, diagnosis, treatment and discharge of their patients." And
> further, "The 1983 Department regulations requiring a psychiatrist to
> supervise diagnosis and treatment of all admitted mental patients are
> therefore invalid.")

Olson, R., Holden, W., Friedman, A., & Faust, J. (1988). Psychological consultation
in a children's hospital: An evaluation of services. *Journal of Pediatric Psychology, 13*, 479–492.

> The authors evaluated records of inpatient consultations at a pediatric
> psychology service and surveyed 77 staff members (physicians, nurses,
> and social workers) on their satisfaction with the service. The most
> frequent patient referrals observed were for depression/suicide at-
> tempt, poor adjustment to a chronic illness, and behavior problems.
> Medically related problems accounted for 46% of all consultations. Ap-
> proximately two thirds of the children were referred for outpatient psy-
> chological services. The service was more likely to follow, on an out-
> patient basis, children with medically related problems. Medical staff
> and social workers indicated overall satisfaction with the service, and
> the level of satisfaction was strongly related to the level of diagnostic
> agreement between physicians/nurses and psychologists. The lowest
> level of satisfaction noted was for verbal and written feedback.

Oregon Health Sciences University. (1985). *Medical staff bylaws*. Portland: University Hospital, Oregon Health Sciences University.

> This document is an example of medical staff bylaws in which psy-
> chologists are included. Articles cited in the document include "Mem-
> bership in the Medical Staff," "Termination of Medical Staff Appoint-
> ment," and "Categories and Privileges of the Medical Staff."

Pallak, M., & Cummings, N. (1992). Inpatient and outpatient psychiatric treatment: The effect of matching patients to appropriate level of treatment on
psychiatric and medical–surgical hospital days. *Applied Preventive Psychology,
1*, 83–87.

> Of 106 patients presenting for inpatient psychiatric admission, 20%
> self-referred, 80% were from hospital emergency or admitting rooms,

only 15% were admitted following on-site psychological evaluation. Those admitted averaged 9 inpatient days followed by an average of 8.5 follow-up outpatient visits. The others were referred for intensive outpatient treatment where they averaged 16.3 visits. One year later neither group had further psychiatric hospital days while those on out-patient treatment had fewer medical–surgical days. Thus, when alter-native treatment resources are available, many hospital admissions are unnecessary.

Pion, G., Kohout, J., & VandenBos, G. (1990). Human resources in mental health. In R. Manderscheid & M. Sonnenschein (Eds.), *Mental health United States, 1990* (DHHS Publication No. ADM 90-1708). Washington, DC: U.S. Govern-ment Printing Office.

The authors provide details on the growth of licensed psychologists by state, noting a total of 56,530 by 1989. Reports on their employment settings. Hospitals were the primary employment setting for 13.9% of 41,260 psychologists (5,735) plus another 454 in HMOs and 42 in nurs-ing homes. Hospitals were the secondary employment setting for 9.1% of 21,373 psychologists (some duplication) or 1,945, plus 85 in HMOs and 21 in nursing homes.

Pope, K. (1990). Ethical and malpractice issues in hospital practice. *American Psychologist, 45*, 1066–1070.

Ethical and malpractice issues arising in hospital practice are re-viewed. Topics include (a) preparation and authorization to carry out clinical responsibilities, (b) personnel procedures, (c) financial and po-litical forces influencing hospital policies, (d) billing procedures, (e) clin-ical procedures for responding to patients' needs, (f) confidentiality, (g) discrimination, (h) internship and training issues, (i) sexual abuse of patients, and (j) staff conflicts influencing patient care.

Rosenheck, R., Massari, L., & Astrachan, B. (1990). The impact of DRG-based budgeting on inpatient psychiatric care in Veterans Administration Medical Centers. *Medical Care, 28*, 124–134.

In 1985 the Veterans Administration (VA) implemented a prospective budgeting system for acute inpatient care on the basis of diagnosis-related groups (DRGs). To assess the impact of this system on psychi-atric care, this study reviewed data on all VA discharges for psychiatric or substance abuse disorders that occurred during the 4 years before and 4 years after this system was implemented. During the 4 years following the implementation of DRG-based budgeting the number of unique patients discharged increased by 15.5%. Average lengths of stay declined by 36.9%, and total annual bed days of care per unique patient declined by 29.7%. These changes occurred in association with an 11.5% reduction in the total number of beds occupied by psychiatric patients, an 8.9% reduction in direct per diem expenditures for psychiatric care nationally, and a 32.7% decline in direct expenditures per episode, after adjustment is made for inflation. Prospective budgeting appears to have had a major impact on the pattern of inpatient psychiatric care in this large health care system.

Sciara, A. (1988). Marketing, management and new perspective and responsibilities for psychologists. *Psychotherapy in Private Practice, 6,* 13–20.

The author suggests that with the increased interest in hospital practice by psychologists, independent practitioners must develop new perspectives of their roles in a hospital setting. Psychologists must understand the pressures on hospitals to develop programs and proposals that will allow them to take advantage of a hospital practice. Psychologists must develop marketing skills to market themselves to the hospitals or to market for hospitals. Along with this expanded practice potential, psychologists must develop new perspectives as business entrepreneurs, managers, and effective members of a system that has not traditionally been open to them. Finally, the responsibilities of working in a hospital system are presented with a view to being accountable to the organization and being able to direct one's activities toward goals that are appropriate for the practitioner and the patient.

Shumaker, S., & Pequegnat, W. (1989). Hospital design, health providers, and the delivery of effective health care. In H. Zube & T. Moore (Eds.), *Advances in environment, behavior, and design* (Vol. 2, pp. 161–199). New York: Plenum.

The authors evaluate recommendations that have been made about ways in which the environment can be improved and consider the reasons that so few have been adopted and tested. They also discuss two implicit models that link sociophysical factors to the well-being of health providers and patients in hospitals; consider potential obstacles to empirically based hospital research and, within this context, the complexity of the hospital design process and the efficacy of patient-based interventions; and examine health-provider-based interventions, exploring issues of the work environment and the provision of care in a hospital setting, and the interactions between nurses and patients. The authors elaborate on two nonexclusive models of hospital design and consider how patient care may be negatively influenced by the impact of the sociophysical environment on health providers. The authors track a "typical" myocardial infarction (heart attack) patient through a hospital.

Silver, R. (1987). New York State: A case study in organizing psychology. *American Psychologist, 42,* 863–865.

An analysis of efforts to organize the directors of psychology at the medical schools in New York State provides an interesting case study of the evolution of psychology's standing in medical school settings. Factors that facilitated this process, and organizational and professional dynamics that impeded it, are discussed. Timidity and lethargy are viewed as major factors that must be overcome in the ongoing efforts to build on what has been accomplished.

Stainbach, R. (1987). Identifying and treating alcoholic medical inpatients: The psychologist's contribution. *Psychology of Addictive Behaviors, 1,* 22–29.

> The author discusses reasons for diagnostic and treatment-related problems regarding alcoholic medical inpatients. Areas of potential contribution by psychologists include (a) increasing diagnostic precision and developing effective intervention strategies through consultation, (b) developing methods to promote patient compliance with treatment recommendations, (c) educating medical staff, and (d) contributing to the research literature. It is noted that the physician's reluctance or inability to diagnose alcoholism is related to personality and attitudes concerning alcoholism.

Steadman, H. (1992, January–March). Predictions of dangerous behavior: A review and analysis of second generation research; and Expert testimony on violence and dangerousness. *Forensic Reports,* pp. 155–158.

> The author comments on articles by N. G. Poythress (see PA, Vol. 79: 29582) and R. K. Otto (see PA, Vol. 79:29580). Studies that examine predictions in inpatient setting should be distinguished from those that focus on community behaviors, threatening behavior should not be included with assaultive behavior as criterion variables, and risk factors should be distinguished from outcome measures.

Stromberg, C. D. (1986). Hospital staff privileges. *Register Report, 25*(13), 9–11.

> The author briefly discusses the practical reasons that make the acquisition of hospital privileges important for psychologists as well as the economic implications of this trend. The parameters within which hospitals may legitimately deny staff privileges to nonphysician professionals are illuminated, followed by a discussion of antitrust action that may be taken when it is evident that such professionals, as a group, have been excluded from hospital membership.

Strumwasser, I., et al. (1991). Appropriateness of psychiatric and substance abuse hospitalization: Implications for payment and utilization management. *Medical Care, 29*(Suppl.) AS77–AS90.

> A total of 539 patient records were examined using standardized utilization review instruments adopted or developed by Blue Cross and Blue Shield of Michigan for determining the appropriateness of hospitalization. Physicians reviewed nurse assessments of the appropriateness of hospitalization for accuracy. Overall, 38% of the inpatient days of care incurred by these patients were unnecessary because the care could have been provided on an outpatient basis. Because outpatient care of psychiatric patients is less restrictive and less expensive, and may be as effective as inpatient care for some patients, these findings point to an important inefficiency in the provision of psychiatric care. Sources of this problem and potential remedies are discussed. Three strategies for reducing the amount of unnecessary hospitalization are increased utilization review and management efforts, the inclusion of

preadmission review, the development and inclusion of psychiatric care in prospective payment reimbursement systems, and the development of psychiatric and substance abuse case management programs.

Tanney, F. (1983). Hospital privileges for psychologists: A legislative model. *American Psychologist, 38,* 1238–1242.

> This article examines closely the legislative process involved in the passage of a bill allowing hospital privileges for psychologists in the District of Columbia. It describes the arguments used by the psychologist proponents of the bill and their representatives, including the benefits to be realized by the general public by competition among health professionals, the education and training of psychologists, and steps taken by psychology itself to identify who among its members is qualified to practice health psychology independently. A cogent analysis of the role of the JCAHO in motivating legislative efforts by psychologists is presented.

Tanney, F. (1985). Hospital privileges, legislation and the political process. *Psychotherapy in Private Practice, 3,* 107–114.

> This article traces one legislative endeavor, the passage of the District of Columbia hospital licensure law, and describes the efforts made by psychologists to secure hospital practice privileges through this law. Specific information on the 20 procedures used to mobilize public opinion as well as obtain access to the legislators themselves is provided.

Thompson, R. (1987). Psychologists in medical schools: Medical staff status and clinical privileges. *American Psychologist, 42,* 866–868.

> It is argued that professional autonomy for psychologists in medical settings requires that psychologists exercise self-governance responsibilities. Inclusion of psychologists on the hospital medical staff is critical because of the self-governance responsibilities afforded to the hospital medical staff by the governing body of the hospital. Central among these responsibilities are the delineation of clinical privileges and the monitoring of quality of patient care. The challenges to psychology inherent in these issues are discussed in terms of the continuing need for political activism and professional "maturity."

Tovian, S. (1991). Integration of clinical psychology into adult and pediatric oncology programs. In J. Sweet, R. Rozensky, & S. Tovian (Eds.), *Handbook of clinical psychology in medical settings* (pp. 331–352). New York: Plenum.

> This chapter discusses the integration of clinical psychology into adult and pediatric oncology programs. Oncology programs in medical settings are important areas of practice for clinical psychologists because of the numerous psychosocial problems secondary to cancer. Identifies these psychosocial problems, offers guidelines for assessment and in-

tervention, and discusses the development and maintenance of the clinical psychology program within the cancer treatment center. Psychosocial issues associated with cancer are quality of life, developmental perspective, and biopsychosocial model.

Wickizer, T., Wheeler, J., & Feldstein, P. (1991). Have hospital inpatient cost containment programs contributed to the growth in outpatient expenditures? Analysis of the substitution effect associated with hospital utilization review. *Medical Care, 29*, 442–451.

> The rapid increase in outpatient expenditures has been the focus of growing attention in recent years. This increase has corresponded with public and private efforts to contain hospital inpatient costs, prompting some analysts to suggest that outpatient expenditure growth is the result of a substitution effect, that is, the substitution of outpatient for inpatient care associated with hospital cost containment programs. Claims data on 43 privately insured groups that adopted utilization review (UR) during the latter part of 1984 or early 1985 were analyzed, comparing outpatient expenditures before and after adoption of hospital inpatient UR to quantify the substitution effect associated with UR. UR was not associated with higher physician office expenditures or with higher outpatient diagnostic expenditures. UR was related to significantly higher hospital outpatient department expenditures. On average, these expenditures were approximately 20% higher ($p = .01$) after the adoption of UR.

Wiggins, J. (1992). Psychological practice in hospitals. *Psychotherapy in Private Practice, 10*, 129–135.

> The author discusses the provision of psychological care to nonpsychiatrically disordered hospital populations. Hospitals have been forced to expand into outpatient and home health care and have called on psychologists to help them in all arenas. The alliance between hospitals and psychologists has been strengthened by psychologists' recent inclusion as independent providers under Medicare. Some areas in which psychologists have proved useful include working with depressed older people, with patients recovering from a serious illness or injury, with those in need of diagnostic techniques, and with potential hospital personnel.

Wodrich, D., & Pfeiffer, S. (1989). School psychology in medical settings. In R. D'Amato & R. Dean (Eds.), *The school psychologist in nontraditional settings: Integrating clients, services, and settings. School psychology* (pp. 87–105). Hillsdale, NJ: Erlbaum.

> This chapter seeks to show that the practice of school psychology in health care facilities is completely appropriate, especially when services are rendered to children. School psychologists' skills match the re-

quirements of many medically related tasks so well that this type of psychologist is often seen as especially valuable and competent. In addition to presenting a rationale for this position, this chapter contains illustrative instances of practices in a medical setting that highlight the potential contribution that school psychology can make in this nontraditional setting.

Wood, K., & Khuri, R. (1985). The psychologist's role in the emergency room: A comparative study. *Professional Psychology: Research and Practice, 16,* 106–113.

> The authors compare evaluations by psychologists, psychiatrists, a psychiatric team, and psychiatric residents of 258 16- to 76-year-old patients in an inner-city hospital emergency room. Neither patient presentation nor medical and psychiatric evaluations varied over time. Other than the finding that psychologists initiated evaluations sooner and hospitalized fewer patients than did psychiatrists, there were no significant temporal or dispositional differences in decisions made between psychologists and the other evaluators. Results are consistent with previous findings that more extensive evaluations lead to fewer recommended hospitalizations. Results also suggest that disposition decisions are affected by training and that psychologists tend to place more responsibility on the patient and the patient's family than do psychiatrists.

Zaro, J. S., Batchelor, W. F., Ginsberg, M. R., & Pallak, M. S. (1982). Psychology and the JCAHO: Reflections on a decade of struggle. *American Psychologist, 37,* 1342–1349.

> Psychologists have been attempting to gain a greater voice in the actions and policies of the JCAHO for more than 10 years. This article outlines the formal and informal attempts that have been made during that period to remove barriers to the hospital practice of psychology. Included are discussions of direct interaction with JCAHO itself, state legislative efforts, the Ohio Attorney General's antitrust suit against the JCAHO, and the Federal Trade Commission's proposed investigation. Attempts to make the JCAHO responsive to psychology's concerns are chronicled, and the gradual changes in JCAHO policies and suggestions of future changes are presented.

Suggested Readings

American Psychiatric Association. (1991). *Manual of psychiatric quality assurance: A report of the committee on quality assurance*. Washington, DC: Author.

Anthony, W. A. (1979). *Principles of psychiatric rehabilitation*. Baltimore: Johns Hopkins University Press.

Ayllon, T., & Azrin, N. (1968). *The token economy*. New York: Appleton-Century-Crofts.

Bellack, A. S. (1989). *A clinical guide for the treatment of schizophrenia*. New York: Plenum.

Berwick, D. M., Godfrey, A. B., & Roessner, J. (1990). *Curing health care: New strategies for quality improvement*. San Francisco: Jossey-Bass.

Deming, W. E. (1986). *Out of the crisis*. Cambridge, MA: MIT/CAES.

Falloon, I. R. H., Boyd, J. L., & McGill, C. W. (1984). *Family care of schizophrenia: A problem solving approach to the treatment of mental illness*. New York: Guilford Press.

Graham, W. O. (1990). *Quality assurance in hospitals*. Rockville, MD: Aspen.

Hersen, M., & Bellack, A. S. (1978). *Behavior therapy in the psychiatric setting*. Baltimore: Williams & Wilkins.

Juran, J. M. (Ed.). (1988). *Juran's quality control handbook* (4th ed.). New York: McGraw-Hill.

Liberman, R. P. (Ed.). (1988). *Psychiatric rehabilitation of chronic mental patients*. Washington, DC: American Psychiatric Press.

Ludwigsen, K. R. (Ed.). (1987). *Hospital practice in California: A manual for psychologists*. Los Angeles: California State Psychological Association, Division of Clinical and Professional Psychology.

Morris, J. A. (Ed.). (1997). *Practicing psychology in rural settings: Hospitals privileges and collaborative care*. Washington, DC: American Psychological Association.

Patterson, G. R., Reid, J. B., Jones, R. R., et al. (1975). *A social learning approach to family intervention*. Eugene, OR: Castalia.

Paul, G. P., & Lentz, R. (1977). *Psychological treatment of chronic mental patients*. Cambridge, MA: Harvard University Press.

Resnick, R. J., Enright, M. F., & Thompson, R. J. (1991). *Guidelines on hospital practice privileges: Credentialing and bylaws*. Washington, DC: American Psychological Association.

Rozensky, R. H. (1991). Psychologists, politics, and hospitals. In J. J. Sweet, R. H. Rozensky, & S. M. Tovian (Eds.), *Handbook of clinical psychology in medical settings* (pp. 59–80). New York: Plenum.

Rozensky, R. H., Sweet, J. J., & Tovian, S. M. (1997). *Psycological assessment in medical settings*. New York: Plenum.

Stromberg, C. D., Haggarty, D. J., Leibenluft, R. F., McMillian, M. H., Mishkin, B., Rubin, B. L., & Trilling, H. R. (1988). *The psychologist's legal handbook*. Washington, DC: Council for the National Register of Health Service Providers in Psychology.

Walton, M. (1986). *The Deming management method*. New York: Doss, Mead.

Additional Resources

Association of Veterans Administration Chief Psychologists (AVACP)

AVACP was formed in 1978 to address professional practice issues and concerns of VA chief psychologists, to ensure the highest quality of inpatient care, training, and research provided by over 1,400 doctoral-level psychologists in the VA. Membership includes chiefs of psychology services in over 150 medical centers and independent outpatient clinics. In addition to publishing a quarterly newsletter for its members, AVACP meets during the APA annual convention to discuss professional and organizational issues affecting the delivery of psychological services in the VA and to promote understanding of the contributions and accomplishments of VA psychologists.

Association of Medical School Professors of Psychology (AMSPP)

Established in 1982, this organization was created to further the research, teaching, and administrative and clinical service contributions of psychologists in medical schools. It promotes the development of appropriate organizational structures and functioning for psychologists within medical schools. AMSPP is concerned with many issues that affect psychologists in medical schools, one of which is the effort of psychologists to secure medical staff membership and clinical privileges in hospitals. The association is now able to provide psychologists who are undertaking revisions of their medical staff bylaws with models and procedural guidelines distilled from experiences of their colleagues in other institutions.

Joint Commission on Accreditation of Healthcare Organizations (JCAHO)

This private, not-for-profit organization was established in 1951 by five national health care organizations—the American College of Physicians, the American College of Surgeons, the American Dental Association, the American Hospital Association, and the American Medical Association—as the Joint Commission on Accreditation of Hospitals. As its purview broadened, so did its title in 1989. The JCAHO conducts voluntary accreditation programs and educational activities for general acute care hospitals, adult psychiatric facilities, drug abuse and rehabilitation programs, alcoholism treatment programs, community mental health services, long-term care facilities, services for developmentally disabled persons, and ambulatory health care organizations. Approximately 7,400 facilities, services, and programs hold JCAHO accreditation, including 75% of the acute care hospitals in the United States. The *Comprehensive Accreditation Manual for Hospitals* is periodically revised and delineates medical staff characteristics. The JCAHO also publishes the *Accreditation Manual for Mental Health, Chemical Dependency, and Mental Retardation/Developmental Disabilities Services.*

Appendix A

Sample Forms

Application for Appointment to the Medical Staff

Name of hospital: _____

Address: _____

Date of application: _____

I herewith make formal application for membership on the medical staff and submit biographical data and declaration as to professional conduct, all duly signed.

Name in full: _____

Office address: _____ Phone: _____

Residence: _____ Phone: _____

Affiliated with (if applicable) _____

Sharing space
joint practice _____

Date of birth _____ Age _____ Birthplace _____

Undergraduate: College or university _____

                  Address: _____

                  Major _____

                  Degree _____ Date _____

Graduate: University _____ University _____

                  Address _____ Address _____

                  Major _____ Major _____

                  Degree ____ Date _____ Degree ____ Date _____

Fellowships or   _____
other graduate   _____
training: _____
(give dates)   _____

Licensure: _____ Number _____

                Has your license to practice in any jurisdiction ever been revoked or suspended? _____ Yes _____ No

Malpractice insurance carrier: _____

Address: _____

Limits of coverage: _____ Expiration date: _____

University appointments: _____

(give addresses and titles) _____

Other hospital staff appointments: _____

(give addresses and dates) _____

IF YOUR ANSWER TO ANY OF THE FOLLOWING QUESTIONS IS YES, PLEASE GIVE FULL DETAILS BELOW OR ON A SEPARATE SHEET OF PAPER.

Has your license to practice psychology in any jurisdiction been limited, suspended, or revoked? Yes _____ No _____

Have you been denied appointment, or renewal thereof, or been subject to disciplinary action by any hospital, professional organization, or military service? Yes _____ No _____

Have your privileges at any hospital ever been suspended, restricted, diminished, revoked, or not renewed? Yes _____ No _____

Has your specialty board status been suspended, restricted, diminished, revoked, or not renewed? Yes _____ No _____

Has your faculty membership in any medical or other professional school ever been subject to disciplinary action or not renewed? Yes _____ No _____

Have you been convicted of any crime (felony or misdemeanor) during the past 10 years? Yes _____ No _____

Do you have any physical or mental condition or substance usage that might limit your ability to exercise the requested clinical privileges? Yes _____ No _____

Have you been hospitalized in the past 10 years? Yes _____ No _____

Have you ever had a professional liability or malpractice claim brought against you that was settled or resolved prior to the initiation of a lawsuit and that involved the payment of funds? Yes _____ No _____

Have you ever had a lawsuit filed against you alleging fraud, professional liability, or medical malpractice? Yes _____ No _____

Experience

Internship: _____ Supervisor: _____

Address: _____ Dates: _____

Internship: _____ Supervisor: _____

Address: _____ Dates: _____

List below all other clinical experience past and present. Give addresses, names of supervisors or colleagues, and dates. Be specific regarding amount of time spent providing individual psychotherapy, group therapy, psychological assessment, and other modalities. Indicate general age categories of clients, including aged, adults, adolescent, and child.

Location	Dates	Experiences
_____	_____	_____
_____	_____	_____
_____	_____	_____
_____	_____	_____
_____	_____	_____
_____	_____	_____
_____	_____	_____

In making this application for appointment to the medical staff, I agree to abide by the bylaws of the medical staff and such rules and regulations that may from time to time be enacted.

I shall conduct myself in keeping with the ethics for practice as outlined by the American Psychological Association with the regulations of the _____ (state) licensing agency for my practice.

It is further understood that continued appointment to the medical staff is contingent on service and participation in the hospital, according to the bylaws of the medical staff.

_____

Signature of Applicant

_____

Date

Recommendations

(This Page for Hospital use only)

Action by Credentials Committee

Date: _____ Signature: _____

Title: _____

Action by Executive Medical Committee

Date: _____ Signature: _____

Title: _____

Action by Governing Board

Date: _____ Signature: _____

Title: _____

Notes

_____

_____

_____

_____

_____

_____

_____

_____

_____

_____

Application for Hospital Privileges

In conjunction with my appointment to the medical staff, I request privileges in the areas listed below. Evidence appropriate to each privilege will be furnished as requested.

	Requested	**Approved**

Patient management privileges:
_____ admit patients   _____
_____ discharge patients   _____
_____ provide, coordinate, and evaluate psychological   _____
      care
_____ write and sign treatment plans   _____
_____ write orders for medical consultation and other   _____
      nonmedical services as needed
_____ supervise staff and trainees   _____
_____ enter consultation notes on charts   _____
_____ other, as appropriate   _____

Clinical assessment privileges:
_____ behavioral assessment   _____
_____ biobehavioral and psychophysiological   _____
      assessment
_____ neuropsychological examination   _____
_____ mental status examination   _____
_____ intellectual assessment   _____
_____ personality assessment   _____
_____ forensic assessment   _____
_____ psychoeducational assessment   _____
_____ vocational assessment   _____
_____ other, as appropriate   _____

Clinical treatment privileges:
_____ individual psychotherapy   _____
_____ group psychotherapy   _____
_____ family psychotherapy   _____
_____ behavior modification   _____
_____ hypnosis   _____
_____ biofeedback   _____
_____ emergency room care/crisis intervention   _____
_____ pain management   _____

Requested	**Approved**

_____ rehabilitation services   _____

_____ other, as appropriate   _____

Consulting privileges:

_____ consultation liaison to other services, as needed   _____

_____ professional development services within the   _____
     facility

_____ program planning and evaluation   _____

OTHER (please specify)

_____   _____

Privileges desired:

Active   _____

Courtesy   _____

Consulting   _____

Affiliate   _____

DATE: _____   SIGNED: _____

APPROVED: DATE _____   _____

    Chairman, Credentials Committee

APPROVED: DATE _____   _____

    Chairman, Executive Committee

APPROVED: DATE _____   _____

    Secretary, Governing Board

Applicant's Authorization and Statement of Understanding and Agreement

For the exercise of the requested clinical privileges, I hereby authorize _____ Hospital, its medical staff, and its representatives to consult with administrators and members of the medical staff of other hospitals or institutions with which I have been associated and with others, including past and present malpractice carriers, who may have information bearing on my professional competence, charter, and ethical qualification. I also consent to the inspection by _____ hospital, its medical staff, and its representatives of records and documents that may be material to and evaluation of my qualifications for staff membership. I hereby release from liability any and all individuals and organizations who provide information to _____ hospital or its medical staff, and I hereby consent to their release of such information.

I understand that the requested clinical privileges, if granted, will be considered to be provisional for a period of 1 year. I also understand that every _____ years thereafter my medical staff membership and clinical privileges will be reappraised and possibly revised.

I understand that additional information concerning my health may be required for the consideration of this application and that my health will be among the consideration reviewed biannually at times of reappraisal for renewal of clinical privileges.

I agree that my activities as a member of the medical staff will be bound by the provisions of bylaws, rules, and regulations of the medical staff of _____ hospital, a copy of which has been provided to me.

When absence or other circumstances temporarily cause me to be unavailable, I will arrange for one or more other members of the medical staff to provide for the continuous care of my patients.

I hereby declare that the statements in this application for clinical privileges and medical staff membership and all attachments hereto are complete and accurate.

Signature of applicant _____

Date _____

Supervision

Patients may be admitted to the hospital only by a health care professional with admitting privileges.

Psychological Assistants

Psychological Assistant: _____

Address: _____

_____

Registration #: _____ State: _____ Date: _____

Supervisor: _____

Address: _____

Is supervisor on staff at hospital? _____

Does supervisor work comparable hours at hospital as assistant? _____

Employer: _____

Address: _____

Employer I.D. number _____

Other professional affiliations: _____

_____

_____

Membership in local psychological societies: _____

_____

Membership in national psychological societies: _____

_____

Membership in international psychological societies: _____

_____

Have you ever been denied membership, or a renewal thereof, or been subject to disciplinary proceedings in any professional organization? If so, give full details on separate sheet.

ELIGIBLE FOR CERTIFICATION: _____ Date: _____

Scientific publications: (Please list)

Psychological/Psychiatric History and Evaluation

All Mental Health Patients

DATE: _____ INFORMANT: _____

1. _____

_____

_____

_____

_____

_____

_____

_____

_____

_____

_____

_____

_____

_____

_____

_____

_____

_____

_____

_____

_____

_____

_____

_____

_____

_____

_____

_____

_____

Name: _____

_____
(signature)

Address: _____

Appendix B

State Laws

Hospital Practice for Psychologists:
State Statutes and Regulations

(States having hospital practice laws as of date of publication)

California
Enacted in 1978; amended in
1980; amended in 1996

Connecticut
Enacted in 1995

District of Columbia
Enacted in 1983

Florida
Enacted in 1990; amended in
1992

Georgia
Enacted in 1983; amended in
1997

Hawaii*
Promulgated in 1992

Iowa
Enacted in 1993

Louisiana
Enacted in 1992

Maryland
Enacted in 1990

Missouri*
Promulgated in 1996

New Jersey
Enacted in 1996

New Mexico*
Promulgated in 1996

North Carolina
Enacted in 1983

Ohio
Enacted in 1991

Oklahoma
Enacted in 1995

Utah*
Promulgated in 1996

Wisconsin
Enacted in 1991

Sample Language of Laws (for illustrative purposes only)

California

§1316.5 Clinical psychologists; appointment; use of facilities
(a) The rules of a health facility may enable the appointment of clinical psychologists on such terms and conditions as the facility shall establish. In such health facilities, clinical psychologists may hold membership and serve on committees of the medical staff and carry professional responsibilities consistent with the scope of their licensure and their competence, subject to the rules of the health facility.

Nothing in this section shall be construed to require a health facility to offer a specific health service or services not otherwise offered. If a

---

*Regulations

health service is offered by a health facility with both licensed physicians and surgeons and clinical psychologists on the medical staff, which both licensed physicians and surgeons and clinical psychologists are authorized by law to perform, such service may be performed by either, without discrimination.

This subdivision shall not prohibit a health facility which is a clinical teaching facility owned or operated by a university operating a school of medicine from requiring that a clinical psychologist have a faculty teaching appointment as a condition for eligibility for staff privileges at that facility.

In any health facility providing staff privileges to clinical psychologists, the health facility staff processing, reviewing, evaluating, and determining qualifications for staff privileges for medical staff shall include, if possible, staff members who are clinical psychologists.

(b) No classification of health facilities by the state department, nor any other classification of heath facilities based on quality of service or otherwise, by any person, body, or governmental agency of this state or any subdivision thereof, shall be affected by a health facility's provision for use of its facilities by duly licensed clinical psychologists, nor shall any such classification be affected by the subjection of the psychologists to the rules and regulations of the organized professional staff. No classification of health facilities by any governmental agency of this state or any subdivision thereof pursuant to any law, whether enacted prior or subsequent to the effective date of this section, for the purposes of ascertaining eligibility for compensation, reimbursement, or other benefit for treatment of patients shall be affected by a health facility's provision for use of its facilities by duly licensed clinical psychologists, nor shall any such classification be affected by the subjection of the psychologists to the rules and regulations of the organized professional staff which govern the psychologists' use of the facilities.

(c) "Clinical psychologist," as used in this section, means a psychologist licensed by this state and (1) who possesses an earned doctorate degree in psychology from an educational institution meeting the criteria of subdivision (Cc) of Section 2914 of the Business and Professions Code and (2) has not less than 2 years clinical experience in a multidisciplinary facility licensed or operated by this or another state or by the United States to provide health care or is listed in the latest edition of the *National Register of Health Service Providers in Psychology*, as adopted by the Council for the National Register of Health Service Providers in Psychology.

Connecticut

§20-194a. Hospital or health care facility staff privileges allowed

Any hospital or health care facility may allow a psychologist, licensed pursuant to this chapter, full staff privileges in accordance with the standards of the Joint Commission on Accreditation of Healthcare Organizations if the criteria that have been set forth by the hospital or health care facility are met.

District of Columbia

§32-1307 Standards for clinical privileges and staff membership; anticompetitive practices prohibited

(c) No provision of District of Columbia law, institutional or staff bylaw of a facility or agency, rule, regulation, or practice shall prohibit qualified certified registered nurse anesthetists, certified nurse–midwives, certified nurse practitioners, podiatrists, or psychologists from being accorded clinical privileges and appointed to all categories of staff membership at those facilities and agencies that offer the kinds of services that can be performed by either members of these health professions or physicians.

Florida

Chapter 395 Hospital Licensing and Regulation; Part 1—Hospitals and Other Licensed Facilities
§395.002 Definitions—As used in this chapter:

(6) "Clinical privileges" means the privileges granted to a physician or other licensed health care practitioner to render patient care services in a hospital, but does not include the privilege of admitting patients.

(19) "Medical staff" means physicians licensed under chapter 458 or chapter 459 with privileges in a licensed facility, as well as other licensed health care practitioners with clinical privileges as approved by a licensed facility's governing board.
§395.091. Staff membership and clinical privileges.

(1) No licensed facility, in considering and acting upon an application for staff membership or clinical privileges, shall deny the application of a qualified doctor of medicine licensed under chapter 458, a doctor of osteopathy licensed under chapter 459, a doctor of dentistry licensed under chapter 466, a doctor of podiatry licensed under chapter 461, or a psychologist licensed under chapter 490 for such staff membership or clinical privileges within the scope of his respective licensure solely because the applicant is licensed under any such chapters.

(4) Nothing herein shall restrict in any way the authority of the medical staff of a licensed facility to review for approval or disapproval all applications for appointment and reappointment to all categories of staff and to make recommendations on each applicant to the governing board, including the delineation of privileges to be granted in each case. In making such recommendations and in the delineations of privileges, each applicant shall be considered individually pursuant to criteria for a doctor licensed under chapter 458, chapter 459, chapter 461, or chapter 466, or for an advanced registered nurse practitioner licensed and certified under chapter 464, or for a psychologist licensed under chapter 490, as applica-

ble. The applicant's eligibility for staff membership or clinical privileges shall be determined by the applicant's background, experience, health, training, and demonstrated competency; the applicant's adherence to applicable professional ethics; the applicant's reputation; and the applicant's ability to work with others and by such other elements as determined by the governing board, consistent with this part.

Georgia

Article 8—Health Service Provider Psychologists
31-7-160 (GCA § 88-3801) "Health service provider psychologist" defined
    As used in this article, the term "health service provider psychologist" means a licensed psychologist who meets the criteria of training and experience as provided in Code Section 31-7-162 in the delivery of direct, preventative assessment and therapeutic intervention services to individuals whose growth, adjustment, or functioning is actually impaired or is demonstrably at a high risk of impairment.

31-7-161 (GCA § 88-3802) Appointment of psychologists to staff of medical facilities and institutions
    A medical facility or institution may provide for the appointment of health service provider psychologists on such terms and conditions as the medical facility or institution shall establish. Psychologists shall be eligible to hold membership and serve on committees of the medical or professional staff and may possess clinical privileges and carry professional responsibilities consistent with the scope of their licensure and their competence, subject to the reasonable rules of the medical facility or institution.

31-7-162 (GCA § 88-3803) Training and experience
    A health service provider psychologist shall meet the following criteria of training and experience:
    (1) The psychologist must be currently licensed by the State Board of Examiners of Psychologists;
    (2) The psychologist must be eligible to be listed in the *National Register of Health Service Providers of Psychology* or have completed not less than 2 years, with 1500 hours each year, of supervised experience in health service of which at least 1 year is postdoctoral and 1 year, which may be the postdoctoral year, is in an organized health service training program;
    (3) A substantial portion of the supervised experience must be in an inpatient setting; and
    (4) Two supportive letters of recommendation from health service providers in psychology who are familiar with the applicant's work must be submitted to the medical facility or institution.

31-7-163 (GCA § 88–3804) Continuation of psychologists currently members of hospital staff or employees

Nothing in this article shall prohibit a psychologist currently a member of a hospital staff or an employee of a hospital from continuing to work in that capacity.

31-7-164 (GCA § 88–3805) Limitation, restriction, or revocation of privileges

Notwithstanding any other provision of this article, the exercise of privileges in any medical facility or institution may be limited, restricted, or revoked for reasons including, but not limited to, the violation of such medical facility's or institution's rules, regulations, or procedures which are applied, in good faith, in a nondiscriminatory manner to all practitioners in such medical facility or institution exercising such privileges or entitled to exercise such privileges.

31-7-165 (GCA § 88-3806) Report of denial or removal to State Board of Examiners of Psychologists

When any health service provider psychologist is denied staff privileges or is removed from the medical or professional staff, such action shall be reported by the facility to the State Board of Examiners of Psychologists.

Hawaii

§11-93-1 Definitions

"Licensed psychologist" means a person who has a doctoral degree in psychology and is licensed by the State Board of Psychology under chapter 465, HRS or is eligible for licensure and obtains licensure within 2 years of employment as provided for in chapter 465, HRS.

"Medical staff" means physicians, dentists, podiatrists and other individuals licensed by the state, who are permitted by law and who have been authorized by the governing body to provide patient care services within the facility. All medical staff members and other individuals who are permitted by law and by the hospital to provide patient care services independently in the hospital shall have delineated clinical privileges that allow them to provide patient care services within the scope of their clinical privileges.

Iowa

135B.7. Rules and enforcement

The department, with the advice and approval of the hospital licensing board and approval of the state board of health, shall adopt rules setting out the standards for the different types of hospitals to be licensed under this chapter. The department shall enforce the rules. Rules or standards shall not be adopted or enforced which would have the effect of denying a license to a hospital or other institution required to be licensed, solely by reason of the school or system of practice employed or permitted to be employed by physicians in the hospital, if the school or system of practice is recognized by the laws of this state.

The rules shall state that a hospital shall not deny clinical privileges to physicians and surgeons, podiatrists, osteopaths, osteopathic surgeons, dentists, or certified health service providers in psychology licensed under chapter 148, 149, 150, 150A, or 153, or section 154B.7 solely by reason of the license held by the practitioner or solely by reason of the school or institution in which the practitioner received medical schooling or post-graduate training if the medical schooling or postgraduate training was accredited by an organization recognized by the council on postsecondary accreditation or an accrediting group recognized by the United States Department of Education. A hospital may establish procedures for interaction between a patient and a practitioner. Nothing in the rules shall prohibit a hospital from limiting, restricting, or revoking clinical privileges of a practitioner for violation of hospital rules, regulations, or procedures established under this paragraph, when applied in good faith and in a non-discriminatory manner. Nothing in this paragraph shall require a hospital to expand the hospital's current scope of service delivery solely to offer the services of a class of providers not currently providing services at the hospital. Nothing in this section shall be construed to require a hospital to establish rules which are inconsistent with the scope of practice established for licensure of practitioners to whom this paragraph applies. This section shall not be construed to authorize the denial of clinical privileges to a practitioner or class of practitioners solely because a hospital has as employees of the hospital identically licensed practitioners providing the same or similar services.

The rules shall require that a hospital establish and implement written criteria for the granting of clinical privileges. The written criteria shall include but are not limited to consideration of the ability of an applicant for privileges to provide patient care services independently and appropriately in the hospital; the license held by the applicant to practice; training, experience, and competence of the applicant; and the relationship between the applicant's request for the granting of privileges and the hospital's current scope of patient care services, as well as the hospital's determination of the necessity to grant privileges to a practitioner authorized to provide comprehensive, appropriate and cost-effective services.

The department shall adopt rules requiring hospitals to establish and implement protocols for responding to the needs of patients who are victims of domestic abuse, as defined in section 236.2.

Louisiana

§2114 Organization of medical and dental staff

A. Each hospital shall have a single, organized medical and dental staff. Medical and dental staff membership shall include doctors of medicine or osteopathy who are currently licensed to practice medicine or osteopathy by the Louisiana State Board of Medical Examiners and dentists licensed to practice dentistry by the Louisiana State Board of Dentistry.

B. Each hospital offering care or services within the scope of the practice of psychology, as defined in R.S. 37:2352(5), prior to January 1, 1993, shall establish rules, regulations, and procedures for consideration of an application for medical staff membership and clinical privileges submitted by a psychologist licensed to practice psychology by the Louisiana State Board of Examiners of Psychologists. No hospital shall deny such medical staff membership and clinical privileges solely because the applicant is licensed under R.S. 37:2351 et seq.

C. No individual shall be automatically entitled to membership on the medical and dental staff or to the exercise of any clinical privilege solely on the basis of his license to practice in any state, his membership in any professional organization, his certification by any clinical examining board, or his clinical privileges or staff membership at another hospital without meeting the reasonable criteria for membership established by the governing body of the respective hospital.

D. The provisions of this section shall in no way affect the provisions of R.S. 37:1301.

E. A hospital shall establish rules, regulations and procedures setting forth the nature, extent and type of staff membership and clinical privileges, as well as the limitations placed by the hospital on said staff membership and clinical privileges for all health care providers practicing therein.

Maryland

§19-351 Staff

(d) Licensed psychologists. (1) A hospital or related institution that provides services of the type that licensed psychologists are permitted to perform under Title 18 of the Health Occupations Article shall include in its bylaws, rules or regulations, provisions for use of facilities by and staff privileges for qualified psychologists.

(2) The hospital or related institution may restrict use of facilities and staff privileges by psychologists to those psychologists who meet the qualifications that the hospital or related institution sets for granting those privileges.

(3) (I) Nothing in this subsection shall be construed to require a hospital to:

1. Grant admitting privileges to a psychologist; or

2. Permit the exercise of those privileges granted by the hospital board of trustees to psychologists without appropriate collaboration with the physician who has privileges to admit and attend patients in the unit of the facility where the patient is being treated and who has ongoing responsibility for the patient.

(ii) In the event of a disagreement between the psychologist and the physician concerning the patient's treatment, the decision of the physician who has ongoing responsibility shall govern.

Missouri

(C) Medical Staff

1. The medical staff shall be organized, shall develop and, with the approval of the governing body, shall adopt bylaws, rules, and policies governing their professional activities in the hospital.

2. Medical staff membership shall be limited to physicians, dentists, psychologists, and podiatrists. They shall be currently licensed to practice their respective professions in Missouri. The bylaws of the governing body and medical staff shall include the procedure to be used in processing applications for medical staff membership; approving or disapproving appointments; and determining the privileges available to physicians, dentists, psychologists, and podiatrists.

3. No application for membership on the medical staff shall be denied based solely on the applicant's professional degree or the school or health care facility in which the practitioner received medical, dental, psychology or podiatry schooling, postgraduate training or certification, if the schooling or postgraduate training for a physician was accredited by the American Medical Association or the American Osteopathic Association, for a dentist was accredited by the American Dental Association's Commission on Dental Accreditation, for a psychologist was accredited with accordance to Chapter 337, RSMo and for a podiatrist was accredited by the American Podiatric Medical Association. Each application for staff membership shall be considered on an individual basis with objective criteria applied equally to each applicant.

4. Each physician, dentist, psychologist, or podiatrist requesting staff membership shall submit a written application to the chief executive officer of the hospital on a form approved by the governing body. Each application shall be accompanied by evidence of education, training, professional qualifications, license and standards of performance.

5. The governing body, acting upon recommendations of the medical staff, shall approve or disapprove appointments. Written criteria shall be developed for privileges extended to each member of the staff. A formal mechanism shall be established for recommending to the governing body delineation of privileges, curtailment, suspension or revocation of privileges and appointment or reappointment to the medical staff. The mechanism shall include an inquiry of the National Practitioner Data Bank.

New Jersey

26:2H-12.1 Podiatrists, psychologists; use of facilities

a. Any health care facility licensed pursuant to P.L.1971, c. 136 (C. 26:2H-1 et seq.), which provides medical or surgical care, shall provide for the use of the facility by, and appropriate privileges for, duly licensed podiatrists and psychologists. Use of the facility and privileges of a podiatrist or psychologist shall be subject to nondiscriminatory rules and regulations governing such use or privileges established by the governing body of the facility for persons licensed as physicians and surgeons pursuant to R.S. 45:9-6 and dentists pursuant to R.S. 45:6-19.

b. Nothing in this act shall be construed to require a hospital to grant admitting privileges to a psychologist or to permit the exercise of those privileges granted by the hospital without appropriate collaboration with the attending physician of the patient who is receiving or will receive care or treatment from the psychologist.

Amended by L.1995, c. 310, § 1, eff. Jan. 5, 1996.

New Mexico

106. Definitions
K. "Medical staff" means the hospital's organized component of physicians, podiatrists, dentists, and psychologists appointed by the governing body of the hospital and granted specific privileges for the purpose of providing adequate medical, podiatric, and dental care for the patients of the hospital.

107. Required Licensure by the Department
F. Medical Staff Appointments. The governing body shall appoint members of the medical staff in accordance with the approved medical staff by-laws.

1. A formal procedure shall be established, governed by written rules covering application for medical staff membership and the method of processing an application;

2. The procedure related to the submission and processing of applications shall involve the chief executive officer, the credentials committee of the medical staff or its counterpart, and the governing body;

3. Selection of physicians, dentists, podiatrists, and psychologists and definition of their medical, dental, pediatric, or psychological privileges, both for new appointments and reappointments, shall be based on written criteria;

4. Action taken by the governing body on applications for medical staff appointments shall be in writing;

5. Written notification of applicants shall be made by either the governing body or its designated representative;

6. Applicants selected for medical staff appointment shall sign an agreement to abide by the medical staff rules and by-laws; and

7. The governing body shall establish a procedure for appeal and hearing by the governing body or a designated committee if the applicant or the medical staff wishes to contest the decision on an application for medical staff appointments.

H. Patient Care. The governing body shall establish a policy which requires that every patient be under the care of a physician, dentist, podiatrist, or psychologist. The policy shall provide that:

1. A person may be admitted to a hospital only on the recommendation of a physician, dentist, podiatrist, or psychologist, with a physician designated to be responsible for the medical aspects of care;

2. A member of the house staff or another physician shall be on duty or on call at all times.

300. Medical Staff
c. Membership.

1. *Active Staff.* Regardless of any other categories of medical staff having privileges in the hospital, a hospital shall have an active staff which performs all the organizational duties pertaining to the medical staff. Active staff membership shall be limited to individuals who are currently licensed to practice medicine, osteopathic medicine, podiatric medicine, dentistry, or psychology. These individuals may be granted membership in accordance with the medical staff by-laws and rules, and in accordance with the bylaws of the hospital. A majority of the members of the active staff shall be physicians.

2. *Other Staff.* The medical staff may include one or more categories defined in the medical staff by-laws in addition to the active staff.

North Carolina

§131E-85. Hospital privileges and procedures
    (a) The granting or denial of privileges to practice in hospitals to physicians licensed under Chapter 90 of the General Statutes, Article 1, dentists and podiatrists and the scope and delineation of such privileges shall be determined by the governing body of the hospital. Such determinations shall be based upon the applicant's education, training, experience, demonstrated competence and ability, and judgment and character of the applicant, and the reasonable objectives and regulations of the hospital, including but not limited to appropriate utilization of hospital facilities, in which privileges are sought. Nothing in this Part shall be deemed to mandate hospitals to grant or deny to any such individuals or others privileges to practice in hospitals.

Ohio

3701.351 Hospital staff and professional privileges; procedures; discrimination prohibited
    (A) The governing body of every hospital shall set standards and procedures to be applied by the hospital and its medical staff in considering and acting upon applications for staff membership or professional privi-

leges. These standards and procedures shall be available for public inspection.

(B) The governing body of any hospital, in considering and acting upon applications for staff membership or professional privileges within the scope of the applicants' respective licensure, shall not discriminate against a qualified person solely on the basis of whether that person is certified to practice medicine, osteopathic medicine, or podiatry, or licensed to practice dentistry or psychology. Staff membership or professional privileges shall be considered and acted on in accordance with standards and procedures established under division (A) of this section. This section does not permit a psychologist to admit a patient to a hospital in violation of section 3727.06 of the revised code.

(C) The governing body of any hospital that is licensed to provide maternity services, in considering and acting upon applications for clinical privileges, shall not discriminate against a qualified person solely on the basis that the person is certified to practice nurse–midwifery. An application from a nurse–midwife shall contain the name of a physician member of the hospital's medical staff who holds clinical privileges in obstetrics at that hospital and who has agreed to direct and supervise the applicant in accordance with section 4723.43 of the Revised Code.

(D) Any person may apply to the court of common pleas for temporary or permanent injunctions restraining a violation of division (A), (B), or (C) of this section. This action is an additional remedy not dependent on the adequacy of the remedy at law.

(E)(1) If a hospital does not provide or permit the provision of any diagnostic or treatment service for mental or emotional disorders or any other service that may be legally performed by a psychologist licensed under chapter 4732 of the Revised Code, this section does not require the hospital to provide or permit the provision of any such service and the hospital shall be exempt from requirements of this section pertaining to psychologists.

(2) This section does not impair the right of a hospital to enter into an employment, personal service, or any other kind of contract with a licensed psychologist, upon any such terms as the parties may mutually agree, for the provision of any service that may be legally performed by a licensed psychologist.

Oklahoma

§1-707a. Staff privileges–Applications–Psychologists

A. The administrator in charge of each hospital or related institution licensed by the state Commissioner of Health shall accept for consideration each application for professional staff privileges submitted by a person licensed to practice:

1. Medicine by the State Board of Medical Licensure and Supervision;
2. Osteopathy by the State Board of Osteopathy;
3. Podiatry by the State Board of Podiatry; or

4. As a health service psychologist by the Oklahoma State Board of Examiners of Psychologists.

B. The Application shall be acted upon by the governing board of the hospital within a reasonable time. A written report of such action shall be furnished to the applicant thereafter.

C. If a hospital grants staff privileges to a psychologist, at the time of admission of a patient of a psychologist to the hospital, the psychologist or the hospital shall identify a psychiatrist, a medical doctor, or a doctor of osteopathy who shall be responsible for the evaluation and medical management of the patient.

Utah

R432. Health, Health Systems Improvement, Health Facility Licensure.
R432-100. General Hospital Standards.
R432-100-6. Medical and Professional Staff.

(1) Organization

(a) Each hospital shall have an organized medical staff that operates under bylaws approved by the board and is responsible for the quality of care provided to patients within the hospital.

(b) The medical staff shall advise and be accountable to the board for the quality of medical care provided to patients.

(2) Bylaws, Policies and Procedures.

The medical staff must adopt bylaws, policies and procedures that address:

(a) The credentialing process including;

(b) The necessary qualifications for membership;

(c) The delineation of privileges;

(d) The scope of privileges for specified professionals who are not members of the medical staff.

(3) The members of the medical and professional staff must be legally, professionally and ethically qualified.

(4) The medical care of all persons admitted to the hospital shall be under the supervision and direction of a fully qualified physician who is licensed by the state.

(5) An applicant for staff membership and privileges may not be denied solely on the ground that the applicant is a licensed podiatrist or a licensed psychologist rather than licensed to practice medicine under the Utah Medical Practice Act or the Utah Osteopathic Medical Licensing Act.

(6) Membership and privileges may not be denied on any ground that is not otherwise prohibited by law.

(7) Each applicant for medical and professional staff membership must be oriented to the bylaws, rules and regulations and policies and agree in writing to abide by all conditions.

(8) In hospitals participating in professional graduate education programs, the rules and regulations and policies specify the mechanism by

which house staff are supervised by members of the medical staff in carrying out patient care responsibilities.

Wisconsin

Uniform Licensure
50.36 Rules and standards

(3g)(a) In this subsection:

1. "Mental illness" has the meaning given in s. 51.01(13)(a).

2. "Psychologist" means a licensed psychologist, as defined in s. 455.01(4).

(b) A hospital that admits patients for treatment of mental illness may grant to a psychologist who is listed or eligible to be listed in the *National Register of Health Service Providers of Psychology* or who is certified by the American Board of Professional Psychology an opportunity to obtain hospital staff privileges to admit, treat, and discharge patients. Each hospital may determine whether the applicant's training, experience, and demonstrated competence are sufficient to justify the granting of hospital staff privileges or of limited hospital staff privileges.

(c) If a hospital grants a psychologist hospital staff privileges or limited hospital staff privileges under par, (b) the psychologist or the hospital shall, prior to or at the time of admission of a patient, identify an appropriate physician with admitting privileges at the hospital who shall be responsible for the medical evaluation and medical management of the patient for the duration of his or her hospitalization.

Appendix C

Sample Indicators

Psychological Assessment

1. The assessment report includes source(s) of data for both background information and the present evaluation.
2. The assessment appropriately addresses referral questions.
3. The interpretation of results is communicated in a clinically useful way with appropriate recommendations.
4. Conclusions, clinical impressions, and diagnoses are supported by test data and other relevant information.
5. An appropriate IQ test and the gathering of appropriate information relative to adaptive behavior are included in assessments when there is a concern about mental retardation.
6. Appropriate tests are administered, and sufficient background information is gathered when specific learning or developmental disabilities are at issue.
7. The formal report is prepared within a specified time period after the completion of the assessment.

Diagnostic Assessment

1. The Assessment Form is complete. If there is need to gather further information in any domain area, there is evidence that this has been completed within (a designated time from) the date of the assessment.
2. The *DSM–IV/DSM–IV–R* Multiaxial Evaluation is complete for all five axes (or *ICD-10-CM* diagnostic system). In the event of a deferred or unknown diagnosis, there is evidence in the record of
   a) a referral for a specialized assessment (i.e., psychological, psychiatric, neurological psychoeducational, psychoactive, substance abuse followed by an updated *DSM–IV/DSM–IV–R* Multiaxial Evaluation or *ICD-10-CM*) or
   b) in the absence of a referral for a specialized assessment, an updated *DSM–IV/DSM–IV–R* Multiaxial Evaluation or *ICD-10-CM* diagnosis is in the record (within a designated time period from the date) of the assessment.

General Treatment

1. Intervention method is consistent with presenting problems.
2. Progress toward treatment goals occurs.
3. Progress is documented.
4. The appearance of or existence of conditions or symptoms that warrant referral for specialized evaluations per the health care facility's clinical procedural manual are accompanied by the appropriate referral.
5. The psychologist is fully privileged in the interventive method used, or otherwise is receiving supervision in relation to it.
6. Changes in treatment focus are documented.

Treatment Plan

1. The date of the most recent treatment plan is not more than a designated time period from the date of the quality assurance review.
2. The treatment plan specifies the problems to be addressed through treatment.
3. The treatment plan specifies the intended outcomes of treatment through goals and objectives that are measurable and are stated in more detail than the opposite of the problem (e.g., stealing vs. not stealing).
4. The treatment plan specifies the interventive methods to be used in a specific rather than general sense (e.g., cognitive–behavioral therapy, assertiveness training, structural family therapy).

Emergency Psychological Assessment

1. Emergency assessments of nonclients are completed by appropriately privileged staff.
2. There is evidence of an evaluation of the mental status of the client.
3. There is evidence in the assessment that a judgment has been made as to the degree of risk of injury to self or others.
4. A diagnosis reflecting the patient's condition at that time is reached and recorded per *DSM–IV/DSM–IV–R* or *ICD-10-CM* typology.
5. The degree and type of social support systems available to the client/family in crisis are reflected in the assessment.
6. The existence of symptoms that are criteria for a referral to or consultation with an appropriate health care provider (per clinical procedures manual) results in the referral or consultation.

Emergency Services and Crisis Stabilization

1. Treatment is provided in a timely manner.
2. The least restrictive treatment program commensurate with the client/family's needs is recommended.
3. The client/family has been given clear assistance and instructions in implementing treatment recommendations.
4. The family's receptivity to the crisis stabilization plan is documented in the clinical record.
5. There is evidence in the record that the proper authorities have been notified when a significant risk of injury to self or others is present and the client/family is noncompliant with treatment recommendations, in compliance with state and local laws and hospital procedures.

Emergency Services and Follow-Up

1. There is documentation in the record of an outreach attempt to re-engage those clients/families recommended for ongoing services that failed to proceed beyond assessment.
2. The outreach attempt is made within a designated time from the date of the assessment.

Glossary

ACTIVITY SERVICES (OR THERAPEUTIC ACTIVITY SERVICES)   Structured activities designed to develop an individual's creative, physical, and social skills through participation in recreational, art, dance, drama, social, and other activities.

ADMINISTRATIVE   Relates to the fiscal and general management of a facility rather than to the direct provision of services to patients.

AFFILIATE STAFF   A category of hospital staff participation defined in the bylaws of facilities that usually includes nonphysician or nondoctoral practitioners in a hospital setting. Rarely do affiliate staff members have full treatment, admitting, and discharge privileges. The affiliate staff status does not usually allow for voting privileges on committees of the professional staff or medical staff.

AFTERCARE   Services that are provided after discharge that support and increase the gains made during treatment.

AP/PF (ACCREDITATION PROGRAM FOR PSYCHIATRIC FACILITIES)   Joint Commission on Accreditation of Hospitals, 875 North Michigan Avenue, Chicago, IL 60611.

APPLICANT   An individual who has applied for admission to a program but who has not completed the intake process.

APPOINTMENTS   The formal granting of membership in a staff category with specific clinical privileges in a hospital.

APPROVED   Acceptable to the authority having jurisdiction.

ASSESSMENT   Those procedures by which a program evaluates an individual's strengths, weaknesses, problems, and needs.

ATTENDING STAFF   A psychologist, physician, or other qualified practitioner who is a member of the organized staff and has privileges to serve as the primary care provider or case manager.

AUDIT, FINANCIAL   An independent review by a public accountant certifying that a facility's financial reports reflect its financial status.

AUTHENTICATION   Proof of authority and responsibility by written signature, identifiable initials, computer key, or other method. The use of a rubber stamp signature is acceptable under the following conditions: The person whose signature the rubber stamp represents is the only one who has possession of the stamp and is the only one who uses it, and this person gives the chief executive officer a signed statement asserting that he or she is the only one who has the stamp and is the only one who will use it.

AUTHORITY HAVING JURISDICTION   The organization, office, or individual responsible for approving a piece of equipment, an installation, or a procedure.

BYLAWS   A formal document that describes how the practitioners of a given hospital are organized. The bylaws include the descriptions of staff categories and the process for application, review, and appointment. The bylaws of a hospital have legal significance for the operation of a facility and the activities of the staff. There is usually a bylaws committee that continually reviews and recommends updating these principles and structures.

CERTIFYING A PATIENT   The process whereby a practitioner determines that a person meets one or more of the criteria for being certified as a patient in need of evaluation or treatment when the individual (patient) is unwilling to so do.

CHIEF EXECUTIVE OFFICER   The individual appointed by the governing body of a hospital to act on its behalf in the overall management of the facility. Other

141

terms used to describe this role include *administrator, superintendent, director, president, vice president,* and *executive vice president.*

CLINICAL PRIVILEGES   Authorization by the governing body to render patient care and treatment services in the facility within well-defined limits, on the basis of the individual's professional qualifications, experience, competence, ability, and judgment.

COMMUNITY EDUCATION SERVICES   The dissemination of information to increase the awareness, receptivity, and sensitivity of the community to the disabilities treated by a facility.

CONSULTANT   An individual who provides professional advice or services on request.

CONSULTING STAFF   A subcategory of the organized staff that includes practitioners who act only as consultants in their fields of specialty. Consulting staff usually do not hold office and are not able to vote in the governance system of the hospital.

CONTINUOUS QUALITY IMPROVEMENT (CQI)   The next generation of quality monitoring after quality assurance. CQI represents the process of evaluating clinicians' activities within the context of the hospital environment. CQI reflects the recognition within the health care industry that quality always can be improved.

CONTRACT   A formal agreement with any organization, agency, or individual, approved by the governing body, that specifies the services, personnel, or space to be provided to, or on behalf of, the facility and the monies to be expended in exchange.

COURTESY STAFF   A subcategory of the organized staff that usually includes practitioners who admit a small number of patients per year to a facility. Often, courtesy staff members do not hold office or vote in the governance system of the hospital.

CREDENTIALING   The process of evaluating a practitioner's training, supervision, and experience by a review of supporting documents.

CREDENTIALS   Documents that support a practitioner's training, supervision, and experience. These materials are used to determine specific staff categories and clinical privileges.

DAY HOSPITAL   An outpatient facility that provides treatment during the day. Patients return home overnight.

DIAGNOSIS   A clinically descriptive statement that identifies the nature and category of a patient's disorder, according to the appropriate diagnostic schemes, such as the *International Classification of Diseases (ICD–10–CM)* or the *Diagnostic and Statistical Manual of Mental Disorders* (4th ed. and revised 4th ed.).[5]

DISCHARGE   The point at which a patient's active involvement with a facility is terminated and the facility no longer maintains active responsibility for the patient.

DISCHARGE SUMMARY   A summary of a hospital patient's history, admission, treatment, and condition on discharge. This summary is required within a specific time, and the form and time limits are monitored by the hospital medical records department.

DOCUMENTATION   The written record of data about a patient's history, assessment,

---

[5]These are the editions of the *ICD* and *DSM* in use at the time of printing. In the event a subsequent version has replaced the editions referenced, the reader should consult the most up-to-date version of the *ICD* or *DSM.*

progress, privileges, treatment plan, and so forth. Justification for hospitalization and proper utilization of the hospital are dependent on specific documentation throughout the patient's stay.

DRG (DIAGNOSTIC-RELATED GROUP)   A patient classification system that is used in the prospective reimbursement system of the Medicare program. For each class, a specific amount of money will be reimbursed regardless of services provided or number of days of care. The system is a matter of great controversy and, in case of mental health care setting, is still in the proposal stage.

DRUG HISTORY   A delineation of the drugs used by a patient, including prescribed and unprescribed drugs and alcohol. A drug history includes, but is not necessarily limited to, the following: drugs used in the past; drugs used recently, especially within the preceding 48 hours; drugs of preference; frequency with which each drug is used; route of administration of each drug; drugs used in combination; dosages used; year of first use of each drug; previous occurrences of overdose, withdrawal, or adverse drug reactions; and history of previous treatment received for alcohol or drug abuse.

DSM–IV (*Diagnostic and Statistical Manual of Mental Disorders*, 4th ed.; American Psychiatric Association, 1994)   This manual provides a categorical system by which behavioral health disorders are classified.

ELECTROCONVULSIVE THERAPY   A form of somatic treatment in which an electrical current is applied to the brain, producing a mild seizure.

EXTERNAL DISASTER   A catastrophe that occurs outside a facility and for which the facility, on the basis of its size, staff, and resources, must be prepared to serve the community.

FACILITY   An organization that provides psychiatric, substance abuse, or mental health services to patients.

FISCAL MANAGEMENT   Procedures used to control a facility's overall financial and general operations. Such procedures may include cost accounting, program budgeting, materials purchasing, and patient billing.

FORMULARY   A catalog of the pharmaceuticals approved for use in a facility. A formulary lists the names of the drugs and information regarding dosage, contraindications, and unit dispensing size.

GOAL   An expected result or condition that takes time to achieve, that is specified in a statement of relatively broad scope, and that provides guidance in establishing intermediate objectives directed toward its attainment.

GOVERNING BODY   The person or persons with ultimate authority and responsibility for the overall operation of the facility.

GUARDIAN   A parent, trustee, committee, conservator, or other person or agency empowered by law to act on behalf of, or have responsibility for, an applicant or patient.

HAZARDOUS PROCEDURES   Procedures that place a patient at physical or psychological risk or cause a patient pain.

HUMAN SUBJECT RESEARCH   The use of patients in the systematic study, observation, or evaluation of factors related to the prevention, assessment, treatment, and understanding of an illness. This involves all behavioral and medical experimental research that involves human beings as experimental subjects.

ICD–9 (*International Classification of Diseases*; Commission on Professional and Hospital Activities, 1978)   This is a three-volume work that lists code numbers for diseases as well as for procedures. Internationally through the World Health Organization and nationally through the U.S. National Center for Health Statistics, the book is the authoritative standard recognized by third-party payers.

INCIDENT REPORTS   Documentation of events or actions that are likely to lead to adverse effects or that vary from established policies and procedures pertaining to patient care.

INDICATOR   A measurement tool for monitoring and evaluating quality of care.

INPATIENT PROGRAMS   Programs that provide services to people who require an intensity of care that warrants 24-hour supervision in a hospital or other suitably equipped setting. Such programs are usually located in facilities classified as institutional occupancies in chapters 12 and 13 of the *Life Safety Code* (National Fire Protection Association [NFPA], 1973, Standard 101).

INTAKE   The administrative and assessment process for admission to a program.

INVOLUNTARY ADMISSION   Admission of a patient to a hospital against his or her will. A legal procedure must be followed, and approved forms must be used for involuntary admission. Identified psychologists in hospitals that are approved to accept involuntary patients can evaluate patients and certify them for involuntary admission. A psychologist may or may not have privileges to formally and independently admit the patient to the facility.

JOINT COMMISSION ON ACCREDITATION OF HEALTHCARE ORGANIZATIONS (JCAHO)   One Renaissance Boulevard, Oakbrook Terrace, IL 60181. An organization devoted to developing national standards of structure, function, staffing, and procedure for health care organizations. Standards are published, and hospitals and other health care facilities request review by the JCAHO. Accreditation is voluntary but carries significant meaning in the areas of public relations, compensation by third-party payers, and perception of quality.

LICENSED PRACTICAL NURSE   A person licensed or registered as a practical or vocational nurse in the state in which he or she practices.

LIFE SAFETY CODE (NFPA, 1973)   A set of standards by licensing agencies to assure that a facility meets appropriate physical safety requirements.

LISTED   Used to indicate equipment or materials included in a list published by a nationally recognized testing laboratory, inspection agency, or other organization concerned with production evaluation. An organization periodically inspects the production of "listed" equipment or materials, and the organization's list states that the equipment or materials either meet nationally recognized standards or have been tested and found suitable for use in a specified manner.

MAY   Used in stating a standard, this word reflects a method of complying with a standard that is minimally acceptable but not preferred. (*See* SHALL and SHOULD).

MEDICAID   A federal program that provides medical services to the financially and medically needy through grants to states. Administered by the Health Care Financing Administration (HCFA) under the U.S. Department of Health and Human Services (HHS).

MEDICAL RECORD TECHNICIAN, QUALIFIED   An accredited record technician who has successfully passed the appropriate accreditation examination conducted by the American Medical Record Association or who has the documentation equivalent in education, training, or experience.

MEDICAL STAFF   A formal organization of practitioners with the delegated responsibility and authority to maintain proper standards of hospital care and to plan for continued betterment of that care. This organization includes qualified independent practitioners such as psychologists, physicians, oral surgeons, or podiatrists as may be specified in state law. (*See also* PROFESSIONAL STAFF.)

MEDICARE   A federal program that provides basic health benefits to recipients of social security through the Social Security Trust Fund. Administered by HCFA under HHS.

MULTIDISCIPLINARY TEAM   A group of clinical staff members composed of representatives from different professions, disciplines, or service areas.

OBJECTIVE   An expected result or condition that takes less time to achieve than a goal, is stated in measurable terms, has a specified time for achievement, and is related to the attainment of a goal.

OCCUPATIONAL THERAPIST, QUALIFIED   An individual who is a graduate of an occupational therapy program approved by a nationally recognized accrediting body, or who currently holds certification by the American Occupational Therapy Association as a registered occupational therapist, or who has the documented equivalent in education, training, or experience; who meets current legal requirements of licensure or registration; and who is currently competent in the field.

OCCURRENCE SCREENING   The process of monitoring selected points in the treatment process.

ORGANIZED STAFF   (*See* PROFESSIONAL STAFF.)

OUTPATIENT PROGRAMS   Programs that provide services to people who generally do not need the level of care associated with the more restrictive environments of inpatient or residential programs. Such programs are usually located in facilities classified as business occupancies in chapter 13 of the *Life Safety Code* (NFPA, 1973, Standard 101).

OUTREACH   The process of systematically interacting with the community to identify people in need of services, to alert people and their families to the availability of services, to locate needed services, and to enable people to enter the service delivery system.

PARTIAL HOSPITALIZATION PROGRAMS   Programs that provide services to people who generally do not require the level of care provided in the more restrictive environment of residential or inpatient programs. Partial hospitalization programs are designed for patients who spend only part of a 24-hour period in the facility; they provide sleeping accommodations that are usually located in the facilities classified as residential occupancies in chapter 11 of the *Life Safety Code* (NFPA, 1973, Standard 101), and they provide treatment and care services only during the day and are usually located in facilities classified as business occupancies in chapter 13 of the *Life Safety Code*.

PATIENT   An individual who receives treatment services. The word *patient* is synonymous with *client, resident, consumer,* and *recipient* of treatment services.

PEER REVIEW   A service provided by professional associates to assess treatment goals and processes and to establish for the payer that treatment is medically or psychologically necessary and appropriate.

PERSONNEL RECORD   The complete employment record of a staff member or an employee, including job application, education and employment history, performance evaluation, and, when applicable, evidence of current licensure, certification, or registration.

PHARMACIST   An individual who has a degree in pharmacy and is licensed and registered to prepare, preserve, compound, and dispense drugs and chemicals in the state in which he or she practices and competent to review all prescriptions being used by a patient for any incompatibility or other counterindications.

PHYSICIAN, QUALIFIED   A doctor of medicine or a doctor of osteopathy who is fully licensed to practice medicine in the state in which he or she practices.

PRACTITIONER   Any person licensed to perform specific treatment for fees, including psychologists, psychiatrists, physicians, dentists, and podiatrists.

PRIMARY PRACTITIONER   The professional who has primary responsibility for the treatment and management of a hospital patient. This person usually writes the orders for and admits and discharges patients.

PRIVILEGING   The process of evaluating an individual practitioner's professional qualifications, experience, competence, ability, and judgment for the purpose of granting the practitioner specific clinical privileges.

PROFESSIONAL STAFF   A more recent term than *medical staff* that is multidisciplinary and describes the organization of professionals delegated the responsibility and authority to maintain proper standards of hospital care and to plan for the continued improvement of that care. This is often a medical staff that has been expanded to include professionals who are nonphysicians. (*See also* MEDICAL STAFF.)

PROGRAM   A general term for an organized system of services designed to address the needs of patients.

PROGRAM EVALUATION   An assessment component of a facility that determines the degree to which a program is meeting its stated goals and objectives.

PROGRESS NOTE   A specific documentation about the treatment and response of a patient in the hospital.

PROSPECTIVE PAYMENT SYSTEM (PPS)   A system used to establish in advance the rate at which a service will be reimbursed, for example, on the basis of an assigned DRG. (*See also* DRG.)

PROVISIONAL APPOINTMENT   Most privileges or new staff appointments are granted on a provisional basis for a specific time. During this time, the credentials committee and other staff members can review the performance of the provisional member. At the end of the time period, a decision is made to move the practitioner to regular status in one of the staff categories.

PSYCHIATRIC HEALTH FACILITY   A specialty category of licensed health facility. A psychiatric health facility is defined in California law as one that provides acute 24-hour inpatient care for mentally disordered, incompetent, or other persons as described in Division 5 or 6 of the Welfare and Institutions Code.[6] Such care shall include, but is not limited to, the following basic services: psychiatry, clinical psychology, psychiatric nursing, social work, rehabilitation, drug administration, and food service. Patients whose physical health needs cannot be met on an outpatient basis must be transferred to an affiliated hospital.

PSYCHIATRIC NURSE, QUALIFIED   A licensed nurse who has a master's degree in nursing, or who has been certified to practice psychiatric nursing by the voluntary certification process of the American Nurses' Association, or who has the documented equivalent in education, training, or experience.

PSYCHIATRIST, QUALIFIED   A doctor of medicine who specializes in the assessment and treatment of individuals having psychiatric disorders, and who is fully licensed to practice medicine in the state in which he or she practices.

PSYCHOLOGIST   As used herein, a psychologist is a person (a) who is licensed or certified as a psychologist, at the independent practice level, by the state in which the psychologist practices; (b) who holds a doctorate degree from a graduate psychology program that is regionally accredited or accredited by the APA; and (c) who has at least 2 years of supervised experience, at least 1 of which is postdoctoral.

QUALITY ASSURANCE (QA)   A system of measuring treatment quality that evaluates the activities of the individual clinician seeking to identify instances of sub-

---

[6]The Psychiatric Health Facility is defined in California's *Health and Safety Code*, Section 1250-2.

standard care. QA is gradually being replaced by more modern methodologies because of its failure to consider the interaction of clinicians with the surrounding hospital environment and because of the recognition that quality cannot be guaranteed, only improved.

REGISTERED NURSE   A person licensed and registered to practice nursing in the state in which he or she practices, who often possesses a baccalaureate degree.

RESIDENTIAL TREATMENT PROGRAM   Programs that provide services to people who require a less restrictive environment than an acute inpatient program and who are capable of self-preservation during an internal disaster. Such programs are usually located in facilities classified as residential occupancies in chapter 11 of the *Life Safety Code* (NFPA, 1973, Standard 101).

RESTRAINT   A physical or mechanical device used to restrict the movement of the whole or a portion of a patient's body. This does not include mechanisms used to assist a patient in obtaining and maintaining normative body functioning (e.g., braces and wheelchairs).

RULES AND REGULATIONS   A document that specifically (or operationally) describes the implementation of the principles established in the hospital staff bylaws. Such issues as procedures for admission and discharge of patients and the content and form of patients' health records are described in the rules and regulations. (*See also* BYLAWS.)

SECLUSION   A procedure that isolates a patient to a specific environmental area removed from the patient community.

SERVICE   Defines a functional division of professional service within a hospital as an organization. Some services are psychology, internal medicine, neurology, pediatrics, rehabilitation medicine, and psychiatry.

SHALL   Used in stating a standard, this word indicates that complying with a standard is mandatory.

SHOULD   Used in stating a standard, this word indicates the commonly accepted method of complying to standard.

SOCIAL ASSESSMENT   The process of evaluating each patient's environment, religious background, childhood history, military service history, financial status, reasons for seeking treatment, and other pertinent information that may contribute to the development of the individualized treatment plan.

SOCIAL WORKER, QUALIFIED   An individual who has a master's degree from an institution accredited by the Council on Social Work Education; who has been certified by the Academy of Certified Social Workers; or who has the documented equivalent in education, training, or experience.

STAFF PRIVILEGES   Specifically delineated and granted privileges to treat patients admitted to a given facility. Examples include admitting privileges, individual psychotherapy privileges, hypnotherapy privileges, and group psychotherapy privileges. Privileges are usually requested by psychologists, reviewed by a credentials committee, and granted or denied individually.

STAFF PSYCHOLOGIST   Usually denotes a psychologist who is salaried by the institution. This does not always mean full staff privileges. Note that in California it is not legal for an institution to collect a fee for psychological treatment and to pay staff psychologists a salary. Only the individual practitioner is licensed to engage in fee-for-service arrangements with patients, not a corporation.

SUPPORT STAFF   Employees or volunteers whose primary work activities involve clerical, housekeeping, security, laboratory, record keeping, and other functions necessary for the overall clinical and administrative operation of a facility.

THIRD-PARTY PAYER   Insurance companies, government agencies, or other entities that provide monies for the treatment of physical and mental illnesses for the recipients of treatment.

THRESHOLD   The predetermined point or level at which a significant problem has been identified requiring corrective action.

TOTAL QUALITY MANAGEMENT (TQM)   A management style or philosophy that promotes an organizational culture favoring continuous quality improvement for the benefit of the organization's customers. TQM requires the inclusion of the organization's governance, managerial, clinical, and support staff in the review process.

TRANSFER   Moving a patient from one treatment service or location to another.

TREATMENT PLAN   A formal plan describing the specific goals of treatment and the recommended or planned approaches that may move the patient toward these goals. Hospital treatment plans need to be interdisciplinary.

UTILIZATION REVIEW   The process of using predefined criteria to evaluate the necessity and appropriateness of allocated services and resources to assure that a facility's services are necessary, cost-efficient, and effective.

VOCATIONAL ASSESSMENT   The process of evaluating each patient's past experiences and attitudes toward work, current motivations in areas of interest, and possibilities of future education, training, or employment.

Index

documentation, as term, *142–43*
Dörken, H., 80–82
Dorwart, R., 84
DRGs. *See* diagnosis-related groups
Drotar, D., 82
drug history, *143*
drug usage after discharge, 73
DSM–IV. See Diagnostic and Statistical Manual of Mental Disorders
Duckro, P., 89
Dunn, R., 82

effectiveness of care, 66
Eisenberg, M., 82
elderly patients, 86–87
electroconvulsive therapy, *143*
emergency psychiatry, 86
emergency psychological assessment, 137
emergency room evaluations, 97
emergency services
  crisis stabilization and, 138
  follow-up, 139
Employee Retirement Income Security Act of 1974 (ERISA), 45
Enright, M., 82–83
ethical issues, 24, 71, 92
Ethical Principles (APA, 1992), 24, 71
examinations. *See* medical examinations; mental status examinations
external disaster, *143*

facility, *143*
Faust, J., 91
Federal Employee Health Benefit Plan, 53–54
federal law, 53–54. *See also* legislative change; state law
  recognition of psychologists, 48–49
  state jurisdiction and, 45, 54
Feldstein, P., 96
Fenton, L., 79
financial audit, *141*
fiscal management, *143*
Fisher, W., 84
flexibility, 36
Florida, hospital practice law in, 119–120
FOC laws. *See* freedom of choice laws
Follette, W., 84
forensic psychology, 11–12
forms, samples of
  appointment to the medical staff form, 105–06
  experience listing form, 107
  psychological/psychiatric history and evaluation form, 113

recommendations form, 108
request for hospital privileges form, 109–110
supervision form, 112
formulary, *143*
freedom of choice (FOC) laws, 49
frequency of treatment performance measures, 73
Friedman, A., 91

Garrick, T., 84
General Guidelines (APA, 1992), 24
Georgia, hospital practice law in, 120–21
Ginsberg, M. R., 97
goal, *143*
  quality improvement programs and, 62
  treatment and, 31, 73
Goldsmith, L., 85
Goldwurm, G., 84
Goodman, J., 77, 85
governing body, 13–14, *143*
graduate education and training, 9–12, 89
group interventions, 11, 84
guardian, *143*
Gutmann, M., 85

Hawaii, 81, 121
hazardous procedures, *143*
HCFA. *See* Health Care Financing Administration
health care advisory committees, 51
Health Care Financing Administration (HCFA), 54, 62
health maintenance organizations (HMOs), 39, 45
Hester, R., 90
Hickling, E., 85–86
history, 29
HMOs. *See* health maintenance organizations
Holden, W., 91
Holmes, J., 86
Holtz, J., 85–86
honorary organized staff, 20
Hopkin, J., 86
hospital administrator, 14, 43
hospital bylaws, 15–16, 91
  model language for, 24
hospital culture, 24–36
  billing, 28–29
  documentation requirements, 29–34
  medical concerns and, 26–27
  on-call requirements, 28
  role relationships in, 36